The Encyclopedia of Nursing Care Quality
Volume I

Issues and Strategies for Nursing Care Quality

The Encyclopedia
of Nursing Care Quality

Volume I — Issues and Strategies for Nursing Care Quality
Volume II — Approaches to Nursing Standards
Volume III — Monitoring and Evaluation in Nursing

The Encyclopedia
of Nursing Care Quality
Volume I

Issues and Strategies for Nursing Care Quality

Edited by
Patricia Schroeder, MSN, RN
Quality Care Concepts
Thiensville, Wisconsin

AN ASPEN PUBLICATION®
Aspen Publishers, Inc.
Gaithersburg, Maryland
1991

Library of Congress Cataloging-in-Publication Data

Issues and strategies for nursing care quality / edited by Patricia Schroeder.
p. cm. — (The Encyclopedia of nursing care quality : Vol. 1)
Includes bibliographical references and index.
ISBN: 0-8342-0213-1
1. Nursing—Quality control. 2. Quality assurance.
I. Schroeder, Patricia S. II. Series.
[DNLM: 1. Quality Assurance, Health Care—nurses' instruction.
2. Nursing Care—standards. WY 100 I856]
RT85.5I83   1991
362.1'73' 0685—dc20
DNLM/DLC
for Library of Congress
90-14568
CIP

Editorial Services: Ruth Bloom

Library of Congress Catalog Card Number: 90-14568
ISBN: 0-8342-0213-1
SERIES ISBN: 0-8342-0219-0

Printed in the United States of America

1 2 3 4 5

To my husband Steve and daughter Amy
for their love and encouragement

To my parents Irene and Walter
for their faith and guidance

To my family Jeanne, Charles, Michael, Elizabeth, and Timothy
for their friendship and support

Table of Contents

Contributors

Mina Acquaye, BSN, MPH, RN
Nursing Quality Assurance Coordinator
South Community Hospital
Oklahoma City, Oklahoma

Linda M. Arenth, MS, RN
Vice President for Nursing and Patient Services
The Johns Hopkins Hospital
Baltimore, Maryland

P. Mardeen Atkins, BSN, RN
Nursing Quality Management Coordinator
Cleveland Clinic Foundation
Cleveland, Ohio

Mary E. Barna Elrod, BSN, RN
Coordinator
Nursing Quality Assurance
University Hospital
University of Nebraska Medical Center
Omaha, Nebraska

Carol M. Beekman, MSN, RN
Nursing Staff Assistant, Surgery
The Johns Hopkins Hospital
Baltimore, Maryland

Cathy M. Ceccio, MSN, RN
Former Director
Orthopedics/Neuroscience Nursing
Cleveland Clinic Foundation
Cleveland, Ohio

Virginia Del Togno-Armanasco, MN, RN
Coordinator
Nursing Case Management
Tucson Medical Center
Tucson, Arizona

Nannette L. Goddard, MS, RN
Consultant and Lecturer Specializing in
Financial Planning and Management Systems
for Nursing
Houston, Texas

Karen B. Haller, PhD, RN
Director of Nursing Research and Education
The Johns Hopkins Hospital
Baltimore, Maryland

Susan Harter, MBA, RN
Director
Finance, Budget and Staffing
Tucson Medical Center
Tucson, Arizona

Carolyn G. Smith Marker, RN, MSN
President
Marker Systems
Severna Park, Maryland

Mary A. Erickson Megel, PhD, RN
Associate Professor
Parent Child Nursing
College of Nursing
University of Nebraska Medical Center
Omaha, Nebraska

Deborah M. Nadzam, PhD, RN
Project Manager
Indicator Development
Joint Commission on Accreditation of
  Healthcare Organizations
Former Director of Nursing Research
Cleveland Clinic Foundation
Cleveland, Ohio

Diane Fay Puta, MS, RN
Director
Medical Staff Services and Quality
  Management
Sinai Samaritan Medical Center
Milwaukee, Wisconsin

**Mildred Sawyer-Richards, MPH,
  RN**
Director
Nursing Quality Assurance
St. Luke's Roosevelt Hospital Center
New York, New York

Patricia Schroeder, MSN, RN
Nursing Quality Consultant
Quality Care Concepts, Inc.
Thiensville, Wisconsin

Madeline Musante Wake, PhD, RN
Assistant Professor and Director of Continuing
  Education and Outreach
Marquette University College of Nursing
Milwaukee, Wisconsin
Vice-Chairperson, Board of Directors
Trinity Memorial Hospital
Cudahy, Wisconsin

Jo Marie Walrath, MS, RN
Director of Nursing, Surgery
The Johns Hopkins Hospital
Baltimore, Maryland

Jean A. Walters, MS, RN
Assistant Vice President
Specialty Care Nursing
Froedtert Memorial Lutheran Hospital
Milwaukee, Wisconsin

Cathleen Krueger Wilson, PhD, RN
Executive Administrator
Arizona Nurses' Association
President
Specialty Applications
Scottsdale, Arizona

Series Preface

Quality is being touted as the "make it or break it" issue of the decade—a concept that holds true in many aspects of American society. It has, however, become an urgent message in health care.

Quality has been brought to center stage for the nineties. Literature and experience tells us that quality is not only a concern of many—from governmental and accrediting agencies to special interest groups—but it also makes good business sense. The cost of good quality is less than the cost of poor quality. Quality enhances not only the receiver of care, but also the providers of care and services and the very state of the organization. It has been placed at the top of the agenda for organizations, administrators, practitioners, payers, and consumers alike. Quality in health care is being discussed, measured, and actually improved.

The Encyclopedia of Nursing Care Quality, a three volume series, contains descriptions of ongoing work to improve health care quality. Chapters written by noted experts in the field of nursing care quality take traditional nursing quality assurance activities and stretch them with applications of new approaches and refreshed enthusiasm. Recurring themes include the concepts of quality improvement, organizational culture, professional accountability, empowerment of those delivering the work of the organization, and collaboration for quality. It describes not just what is, but also what could, should, and will improve patient outcomes.

Volume I: Issues and Strategies in Nursing Care Quality takes a broad look at quality issues and programs in health care. Chapters include descriptions of state of the art programs to improve nursing care quality. Discussions of excellence in organizations, cost, automation, ethics, collaboration, program evaluation, and nursing QA coordinator roles are also contained in this valuable text.

Volume II: Approaches to Nursing Standards provides an overview of some of the most effective standards models used in today's health care settings. These models have unique features, and are described in relation to not only content and format, but also organizational systems and professional accountability. This text is unique in its ability to provide the reader with enough information to allow comparison and contrast between the approaches described. Other chapters discuss issues relevant to nursing standards including the importance of standards, validating standards, and legal issues in relation to standards. A description of the work of the American Nurses Association and the Nursing Organization Liaison Forum to develop national standards and guidelines is also contained in this volume.

Volume III: Monitoring and Evaluation in Nursing describes real world examples of the use of the ten step process in various specialty practice settings for nursing. "How to" discussions are followed by descriptions of unique features of monitoring and evaluating in different practice arenas such as medical-surgical units, mental health facilities, critical care, and long-term care. Ambulatory care and home care settings are also described. Other chapters discuss monitoring the use of the nursing process, using statistics in QA, clinical interpretation of data, and changing practice. This text provides the reader with many examples and thought provoking issues regarding the monitoring process.

This exciting set of books provides nurses with an overview of where we've been, where we are, and where we're going in the name of quality care. It is gratifying to see progress in a field that remained far too dormant for far too long. But perhaps more exhilarating is the clear message that nurses are making great strides in changing organizations for the wellbeing of patients, and improving the quality of health care for the American public.

Patricia Schroeder MSN, RN
Series Editor

Preface

"The heart of quality is not technique. It is a commitment by management to its people and product—stretching over a period of decades and lived with persistence and passion—that is unknown in most organizations today." (Peters and Austin, 1985, p. 118)

In health care, we have spent years seeking the ultimate technique to demonstrate and possibly improve quality. I say "possibly improve" because health care professionals have been quick to state that almost all we did was as best it could be. Predominantly, our orientation to quality assurance (QA) activities focused on how we could use them to maintain the status quo and show off our good work. QA programs, once described to me as "the ultimate trivial pursuit," have been dogmatic, paper oriented, uninspired, and largely ineffective.

There are several purposes to this book. The first is to broaden the reader's understanding of quality and its pursuit in health care. Quality cannot be neatly defined, and approaches to its improvement cannot be simply described. This book looks at issues that will play a role in QA in the nineties and into the 21st century. Concepts of quality improvement, organizational culture, professional autonomy, automation, collaboration between disciplines, and emerging roles in quality programs all play a part in the quality journey in general, and this book in particular.

A second purpose to this book is to apply these concepts to QA activities found within clinical agencies. Chapters include QA program models and discussions of cost, automation, ethics, collaboration, and communication. Such discussions speak to where quality fits in today's organizations, the dilemmas with which we struggle in integrating it, and perspectives on necessary directions for quality in the future.

The authors who have written chapters are experts and pioneers in the subject. They have forged ahead in the understanding and pursuit of quality and are sharing both the process and the outcome of their struggles. My thanks to these authors for sharing their work.

There is no single correct approach to quality improvement in health care. The years of shifting from one technique to another, from auditing charts to monitoring practice, have yielded an interesting result. Any approach to quality works in some organizations, and likely no approach will work in certain others. We are only now beginning to recognize the many tangible and intangible reasons that create this phenomenon: people, their philosophies, the organizational culture, and the resources that interact to create the end product of quality health care—or not. It is hoped that you will benefit from this book's discussions and perspectives on making quality happen in a clinical agency. If so, the path of the quality journey will have been further illuminated.

SUGGESTED READING

Peters, T., & Austin, N. (1985). *A passion for excellence: The leadership difference*. New York: Warner Books.

Patricia Schroeder, MSN, RN,
April 1991

1

Improving Health Care Quality in the Nineties

Patricia Schroeder, MSN, RN; *Nursing Quality Consultant, Quality Care Concepts, Inc., Thiensville, Wisconsin*

The pursuit of quality in health care is being revolutionized. Quality assurance (QA) activities have routinely evolved in their focus, but they have never enjoyed such attention, recognition, and support.

Quality has become a hot issue for the American public today. Discussions of quality can be frequently seen in popular literature, media programming, and even the daily news. Businesses of all kinds are singing its praises. Quality is being credited for improved worker productivity, decreased business costs, increased numbers of customers, increasing revenue, and a happier and a more committed workforce. The editors of *Quality Progress* magazine ("When Murphy Speaks," 1989, p. 83) summarized the outcomes of quality improvement as revitalization of the economy, improvement of the quality of life, and provision of the experience of the joy of creativity. Quality is being touted as the make-or-break issue of the nineties. Peters states, "Quality and flexibility will be the hallmark of the successful economy for the forseeable future" (Peters, 1987, p. 17). Those organizations that pursue quality with unbridled passion are predicted to be the ultimate survivors. Those who do not will be left in the dust.

Quality-related programs in health care have not historically been as widely supported. QA activities have evolved over time. Precipitated by changing expectations on the part of the Joint Commission on Accreditation of Healthcare Organizations (Joint Commission), QA standards of the seventies focused on chart audits. In the eighties a formal, organization-wide QA program that oversaw the monitoring and evaluation of care was prescribed. Increasing emphasis was placed on participation of all disciplines and departments in the QA program. The movement of QA into the nineties has expanded and gained speed. Emphasis is being placed on quality improvement philosophy, including a personal and organizational commitment to quality, ultimate focus on the needs of consumers, and efforts toward continuous improvement.

Three distinct issues appear to be changing the focus of health care quality programs. While perhaps not all-inclusive, these issues do speak to the evolution of quality programs that we are seeing in some agencies and can expect to see in others. These issues include the definitions used for quality, approaches to the measurement of quality, and the use of quality improvement philosophies.

DEFINITION OF QUALITY

First, the definition of quality and its essential components has broadened. Twenty years ago, it seemed that the quality of health care could be described by the documentation found in patients' medical records. The skills and behaviors of health care providers, as evidenced by such documentation, were considered the ultimate parameters of quality. It has become increasingly clear that quality health care involves much more. It is unquestionable, however, that quality care must begin with educated, skilled, and committed caregivers who are oriented to the expectations for their role within a given organization. Additionally, research-based practice must guide the care of these knowledgeable practitioners.

Batalden suggests that ensuring quality involves meeting the needs of patients, physicians, and payers—three different and essential customer groups (Graham, 1987, p. 24). The needs and expectations of these groups must be determined and measured, and their satisfaction in terms of care delivered ultimately improved.

Patient satisfaction is considered an important quality measure in health care. It is no longer acceptable to deem that a patient received high-quality care if the patient was also dissatisfied with it. Satisfaction with care, once considered only "nice to know," is now both a valid and an essential quality outcome measure, as well as a key variable for the marketing of health care services.

Quality and cost had been considered mutually exclusive issues, but their inter-relatedness is now being recognized. Among studies addressing these issues, Sandella (1990) studied cost and quality in hospitals. Three groups of hospitals were differentiated, based on diagnosis-related group (DRG) denial rates, a cost parameter. Results demonstrated that those hospitals that performed well finan-cially had a strong commitment to quality care. The commitment was demon-strated by staff through the sharing of accountability, "coupling humanistic caring about patients with cost effective behavior by inventing new methods, and fostering teamwork internally and externally" (p. 35).

Available resources also play a role in quality health care. While "more" is not always better, obviously "enough" is necessary. The availability of personnel and wise use of their time play a significant role in today's view of quality. The shortage of many health care provider groups—nurses, physical therapists, occupational therapists, and others—has created quality problems for care deliv-ery in many settings. Hartz et al. (1989) found that hospitals with a high proportion of nurses who are registered nurses provided a higher quality of care, using mortality rates as the measure. The availability of good leaders, educators, and resource people is also necessary in today's fast-paced, ever-changing health care environments. Time, money, equipment—all must be available for quality care to be provided.

The management of risks and the prevention, investigation, and follow-up of errors and accidents are essential parts of quality programs in health care. In today's litigious society, the actual and potential costs, in terms of dollars and human suffering, associated with poor quality are almost unfathomable.

Organizational culture has been considered as having a strong influence on quality. Cooke and Rousseau (1988) define culture as "the ways of thinking, behaving, and believing that members have in common" (Thomas, Ward, Chorba, & Kumiega, 1990, p. 18). Peters and Waterman (1982), Lancaster (1985), del Bueno (1986), Thomas et al. (1990), and even the Joint Commission (1987) all speak of culture as an important component in providing high-quality care. Effective leadership is an essential element in establishing such culture and is thus critical in order for quality care to be provided.

Today's view of quality, then, incorporates knowledge, skills, and behaviors of practitioners, as well as use of patient, physician, and payer measures of quality. Organizational culture, leadership, costs, productivity, and efficiency are also components. Because of this multifaceted vision, the description, measurement, and ultimate improvement of quality are increasingly complex.

MEASUREMENT OF QUALITY

The second issue changing health care quality programs is the measurement of quality. Scientific methods of measurement are increasingly necessary. While QA evaluation does not require the rigorous quantitation that research requires, sound methods are nonetheless necessary to have confidence in the resulting data. Furthermore, data from QA evaluation are being used to create significant change within organizations, so faulty data based on inaccurate measurement methods carry a great risk.

In 1989 the federal government established an organization—the Agency for Health Care Policy and Research (AHCPR)—that will investigate and define outcome measures of quality health care. Several initiatives have begun efforts to pursue the mission of "enhanc[ing] the quality of patient care services through improved knowledge that can be used in meeting society's health care needs " (AHCPR, 1990, p. 1). Both large-scale and small-scale research on patient outcomes is being carried out. Clinical practice guidelines based on the literature are being developed by expert multidisciplinary teams. Other projects and planning are also underway. Such governmental efforts to improve the quality of care will produce major changes in the coming years.

Measurement of quality has decidedly shifted from addressing the process of care to addressing the outcomes of care. This swing of the pendulum has occurred before. Outcome-based evaluation criteria were the foundation of many chart audits in the seventies.

The return to outcome measures has been fostered by many outside of the setting for care delivery. Consumers of health care are increasingly asking what outcomes they can expect from care they have received. Third-party payers of health care are extremely concerned about not simply the care received but also the end results achieved, based on expenses incurred. These payers have identified their own measures of quality outcomes and use them to determine whether full payment should be made. The Joint Commission has moved boldly into the outcome arena, requiring that patient outcome indicators be used for monitoring and evaluation activities (Joint Commission, 1991). Despite their widespread use, though, outcome measures of quality still pose many dilemmas: When does one measure the outcome? To whom can the outcome be attributed? What research-based outcomes can be expected from the implementation of selected interventions? (Hegyvary, 1991). These are but a few of the critical questions about outcome criteria yet to be answered.

In addition to the shift toward outcomes, the Joint Commission has begun development of outcome indicator sets for which mandatory data collection will eventually be necessary. The resulting data are to be used internally within the health care setting, by the Joint Commission on its periodic surveys, and for the development of a national database ("JCAHO: Pilot Hospitals' Input," 1990). It is essential that nurses be well informed of the content of indicator sets under development and support work to incorporate measures that reflect the entire scope of care delivery.

QUALITY IMPROVEMENT

The third issue changing quality programs is the shift from a QA philosophy to a quality improvement (QI) philosophy. Taking the lead from industries outside of health care who have achieved dramatic success in improving the quality of their products and services, some have begun to apply QI principles to health care settings.

The premise of QI is that quality can always be made better. Rather than comparing oneself to a national norm of mediocrity, improvement can only be demonstrated through comparing oneself to oneself over time. QI embodies the message that quality will not be improved simply as a result of inspection. It must be built into the people and the processes carrying out the work of the organization. QI uses workers at the point of service to define quality, measure its achievement, and create innovations to constantly improve. A QI program requires active involvement of all within the organization, from the mailroom to the boardroom. Visible, supportive leadership is essential. Knowledge of and attention to the mission of the organization by all is essential to QI. Collaboration between departments and people, ongoing education, and love of change are all considered critical to the delivery of a quality product or service.

Dennis O'Leary, current president of the Joint Commission, has said, "In retrospect, the word 'assurance' was an unfortunate semantic selection. Quality, of course, could never be assured. Rather it could at best only be improved" (O'Leary, 1990, p. 2). The Joint Commission, in its Agenda for Change, has begun to strongly emphasize the philosophy of QI and has begun to incorporate QI concepts into its literature, standards, and surveys.

REQUISITES TO QUALITY: VISION, APPROACH, CHAMPIONS

Despite these dramatic changes in the view and achievement of quality, its pursuit nevertheless continues to require three essential components: a vision of what quality can be, a dedicated approach to achievement of the vision, and champions to carry out the charge.

The breakneck pace of today's organizations too often leaves us in a reactive stance to change. It may seem that a good leader just maintains the status quo and doesn't rock the boat, but the literature suggests that this could not be further from the truth. The goal and mission of delivery of quality health care must guide a proactive approach to change. An organization's vision of quality must be clear and widely shared throughout the organization.

The approach taken to achieve the vision must be relentless and tireless. It is the rare new program that suddenly makes everything better. QI happens in small steps, through the support and guidance of an organized program and organized leader. The approach must be developed within the organization and must fit with its people, culture, and resources. It cannot be considered a short-term fix or a passing fad, but rather must be supported by an all-out commitment.

Finally, quality programs today can be successful only through the passionate commitment of champions of the cause. Champions of quality must be seen at every level of the organization, and they must be encouraged, supported, and rewarded.

Improving quality will continue to be a major theme in health care as we move into the 21st century. Application of research will guide practitioners to more accurate diagnoses and treatments for patients and their human responses. Care will be guided by scientific data to achieve the greatest efficacy at the lowest possible cost. Health care organizations and systems will be streamlined, and collaboration and efficiency will be greatly improved.

But another wonderful result of the "new" views about quality programs, especially to those of us who have struggled with them in the past, is that these programs are finally being acknowledged as essential to the well-being of the patient, the staff, and the organization as a whole, and that those responsible for the delivery of quality care are themselves assuming a role in improving service. We are finally putting into action something we already knew: that quality comes from people, and people must be prepared, supported, and empowered to carry out their vital roles. As this is further acted upon, we will watch the many potentials of quality and its programs unfold.

REFERENCES

Agency for Health Care Policy and Research. (1990). *Agency for Health Care Policy and Research*. Rockville, MD: Author.

Cooke, R.A., & Rousseau, D.M. (1988). Behavioral norms and expectations: A quantitative approach to the assessment of organizational culture. *Group and Organizational Studies, 13*, 245–273.

del Bueno, D. (1986). Organizational culture: How important is it? *Journal of Nursing Administration, 16*, 15–20.

Graham, J. (1987). Quality gets a closer look. *Modern Healthcare, 17*, 20–22, 24, 27, 30, 31.

Hartz, A.J., Krakaver, H., Kuhn, E.M., Young, M., Jacobsen, S.J., Gay, G., Muenz, L., Katzoff, M., Bailey, R.C., Rimm, A.A. (1989). Hospital characteristics and mortality rates. *New England Journal of Medicine, 321*, 1720–1724.

Hegyvary, S.T. (1991). Issues in outcomes research. *Journal of Nursing Quality Assurance, 5*(2), 1–6.

JCAHO: Pilot hospitals' input updates agenda for change. (1990). *Hospitals, 64*, 50–54.

Joint Commission on Accreditation of Healthcare Organizations. (1987). *A guide to quality assurance*. Chicago: Author.

Joint Commission on Accreditation of Healthcare Organizations. (1991). *Accreditation manual for hospitals*. Chicago: Author.

Lancaster, J. (1985). Creating a climate for excellence. *Journal of Nursing Administration, 15*, 16–19.

O'Leary, D. (1990). President's column—CQI—A step beyond QA. *Joint Commission Perspectives, 10*, 2–3.

Peters, T., & Waterman, R. (1982). *In search of excellence*. New York: Harper & Row.

Peters, T. (1987). *Thriving on chaos: Handbook for a management revolution*. New York: Harper & Row.

Sandella, D. (1990). Cost versus quality: In the balance. *Nursing Administration Quarterly, 14*, 31–40.

Thomas, C., Ward, M., Chorba, C., & Kumiega, A. (1990). Measuring and interpreting organizational culture. *Journal of Nursing Administration, 20*, 17–24.

When Murphy speaks—listen. (1989). *Quality Progress, 22*, 79–84.

2

A Climate for Excellence—
An Impossible Dream?

Cathleen Krueger Wilson, PhD, RN, Executive Administrator, Arizona Nurses' Association, and President, Specialty Applications, Scottsdale, Arizona

The contemporary health care environment is fraught with contradictions. Nurse executives are being told to cut back on expenses while creating new programs to maintain occupied beds, or to be creative and to have a vision but to remain flexible and avoid increasing costs. Can the pursuit of excellence in nursing organizations become a reality in the face of such contradictions. This chapter will address some of the fundamental steps to the development of both a culture of excellence and strategies required for success.

Strategy development will be outlined as a process that produces a roadmap. This roadmap directs a nursing organization's efforts to purposefully move from one point to another. Principles of excellence, steps necessary for achievement, goal definitions, and comprehensiveness of planning will be addressed. Threats and opportunities will be examined in relationship to planning strategies. Finally, the requisite skills for nursing leaders interested in the development of an excellent organization will be discussed, along with a checklist that can be used as a tool for beginning the planning process.

PRINCIPLES OF EXCELLENCE

Peters and Waterman's 1982 watershed work, *In Search of Excellence*, describing the characteristics of organizational excellence, signaled the beginning of a proliferation of a significant body of literature. Over 5 million people have bought copies of this book, which can be taken as reflecting a major transformation of organizational thought! (Peters & Austin, 1985). This thinking has also permeated the nursing literature, as reflected in Kramer and Schmolenberg's (1988b) recent study of magnet hospitals in relationship to excellent organizations.

There are essentially eight organizational principles that predominate in excellent organizations (Peters & Austin, 1985):

1. a bias for action
2. exceptional care of the customer
3. constant innovation through autonomy and entrepreneurship
4. commitment and productivity through people
5. hands-on, value-driven leadership
6. sticking to the knitting
7. simple form and lean management
8. simultaneous loose and tight properties

Are these principles applicable to the health care setting? Can the achievement of excellence be more than lip service—can it be a set of strategic activities purposefully pursued by nursing organizations? Do the current stressors that exist in the contemporary health care environment make the achievement of excellence an impossible dream?

Principle 1: A Bias for Action

This principle is best reflected in an organizational culture that supports experimentation, informal problem solving, and flexibility (Peters & Austin, 1985, pp. 115–197). The latter features are particularly evident in communication and information flow. Traditionally ordered nursing organizations tie information to position rather than to the service process. Yet in order for communication to be effective and meaningful, structures that support a sense of community must exist. This type of environment is a networking one, in which people at all levels constantly share information, resources, and expertise (Naisbitt, 1984, pp. 211–229). The quality assurance (QA) coordinator is a key facilitator in the development and maintenance of such a network. Clearly, communication at the service level is a prime ingredient in the provision of quality care.

Problem solving in excellent organizations is initiated by those individuals who are the most knowledgeable about the problem. The nurse is able to act swiftly and to determine the effectiveness of actions in order to benefit the patient. This action orientation will moderate the normal tendency of people and organizations to conform to the status quo or to be passive. Participation and commitment to professional practice are tremendous in such an environment, further promoting quality patient care.

In order to be knowledgeable, nurses need access to information. Two types of information are required in order to provide excellent patient care: technological/ expert information and knowledge of other contributions to the service process. A lack of information about a patient service will limit successful innovation and problem solving. In addition, ignorance about other contributions to the care process could result in patient care decisions that negatively influence the patient at different points in the process. Such errors occur when one program is funded to the detriment of another. Also, one professional group may eliminate important functions from their job descriptions, without realizing how this decision affects the work at the bedside. Once again, the QA coordinator, who may have a more global view, will be instrumental in providing this kind of information.

Action orientation implies informal relationships. Yet in many nursing organizations, formal bureaucratic structures have resulted in overcontrolled nurse-patient relationships (Porter O'Grady & Finnegan, 1984, pp. 79–105). Such control creates a high potential for negatively influencing quality care. How? Communication cannot be fluid and swift. Necessary patient care information may drop through the cracks or be completely missed because important cues have not been communicated at the proper level. The proliferation of such information management policies benefits management, not the patient, and stifles both nursing judgment and creativity (Porter O'Grady, 1986, pp. 25–42). Such gaps severely limit ability to achieve the full potential for quality patient care outcomes.

An action-oriented environment will minimize such potentials for negatively influencing patient care. In such an environment, problem solving is collaborative and characterized by flexibility, expert authority, and peer relationships. The development of unit-based QA committees is one means of providing an arena for informal problem solving. For example, in a study of 137 hospitals, Cleverley and Stetson (1985, pp. 26–47) found that excellent hospitals were more likely to use expert groups to solve clusters of problems, rather than relying on the typical operational approach.

Magnet hospitals also reflect a bias for action that is characterized by a willingness to experiment, tolerance for errors, fluid communication, risk taking, and futuristic thinking. These characteristics are similar to those found in excellent companies. The nursing culture in such hospitals reflects a strong commitment to patient care and a good deal of trust between nurses and their managers (Lynn, 1990).

Principle 2: Exceptional Care of the Customer

The existence of customer satisfaction programs, which both identify and then evaluate the targeted needs of customer groups, is a hallmark characteristic of excellent organizations. A roadblock in the development of successful customer satisfaction programs in the health care business is the accurate identification of customers and customers needs. The customer is many people in today's health care organization: the patient, the physician, and the insurance company or other payer of health care costs.

Many organizations address the satisfaction of the patient customer via a formal evaluation process. A quantitative approach, based on the administration of satisfaction surveys, is the norm. However, the evaluation of patient satisfaction is, at best, an imprecise science; the questionnaires used to assess patient satisfaction suffer from many limitations. These tools may be outdated and unreliable. For example, the patient needs chosen for evaluation are often determined by administrators or caregivers rather than by patients. This process results in tools that more accurately measure administrators' beliefs about patient satisfaction.

It may be that patient satisfaction is a highly individualized and subjective experience. In fact, in a recent study conducted at the University of Arizona, a qualitative approach was used to measure patients' definitions of satisfaction with care. Patients were asked to describe the behaviors of nurses that instilled confidence. The data of this study are presently being analyzed and will surely provide a basis for a qualitative approach to examining patient satisfaction (Kramer & Schmolenberg, 1988a, pp. 13–24).

Physicians have been recognized as customers of health care organizations for some time now, since physicians bring patients to the hospital, and without patients the organization would not survive. Today, the amount of energy being invested in the physician as customer may be diminishing. Insurance companies are having more and more to say about where patients will be treated. As a result, physicians have been forced to practice at many facilities. In addition, health care organizations have shifted some of the time spent scrutinizing physician satisfaction to determining insurance company satisfaction.

Clearly, insurance companies and managed care programs are nowadays important customers of health care organizations. To not engage in the identification of satisfiers for these customers will result in certain failure. A systematic approach to the identification of insurance company satisfaction is a clear need for organizations interested in attaining excellence. The identification of a standard set of satisfiers for evaluation will be difficult, particularly when an organization works with numerous insurance companies of varying sizes. Universal satisfiers might include (1) the timeliness of communication regarding changes in hospital procedures, (2) a cooperative environment, and (3) the number of inappropriate admissions or procedures and complication/mortality rates. The insurance companies themselves are probably evaluating these and other indicators fairly regularly.

Strategies that target a particular group for enhancement of satisfaction will succeed or fail depending upon the amount and the reliability of information about customer characteristics and expectations for care (Zemke & Schaaf, 1989). QA studies that look at structure, process, and outcome variables together will also yield more complete explanations of excellence in patient care.

Clearly, the advent of managed care programs and a new consumerism has radically changed the how and where of health care decisions. There is a growing recognition that patients and insurance companies must be recognized as groups of consumers, that these groups constitute markets to address, and that these markets have distinct issues and needs (Zemke & Schaaf, 1989, p. 136).

To be fair, it is much easier for a grocery store to produce customer satisfaction than a hospital. The individual nature of health care, the unpredictability of the product, the patient's participation in and observation of the delivery process, and the overvaluation of technology are potential negative influences on satisfaction. For example, grocery stores can stock their products in inventory and check that inventory for flaws, returning damaged goods to the producer. Emergency room services as hospital products are created when the patient arrives at the hospital. The product is highly individualized, depending on the patient's symptoms. Flawed emergency room services cannot be returned. In addition, health care services are chosen *not* by choice but by necessity.

The unique nature of each patient care situation can produce either positive or negative outcomes and challenge the attainment of customer satisfaction. When a blender is purchased, the consumer is guaranteed ahead of time that the equipment will function in a certain predetermined fashion. The same guarantees are not available in health care. Using the emergency room example again, the visit to the hospital is individualized and unpredictable. The predictability of a blender is clearly absent in health care services. The unpredictability of a product can itself negatively influence satisfaction.

Patient care services are not conducive to the commonplace consumer satisfaction tests known as product trials. There is no such thing as a trial-sized pregnancy or heart surgery. Consumer satisfaction in patients is influenced by their expectations of an unknown experience with a health care services product. In fact, health care organizations are most often confronted with unwilling consumers of their product.

The patient's participation in the actual production process is paramount in most health care services. The patient must participate in the delivery of care, cooperating with even the most painful of procedures. This variable also influences consumer satisfaction in patients. Flaws in the production process, such as long waits in the emergency room, are readily observed by the consumer of the services at the time of purchase. In the grocery store example, the customer has no contact with the production process. It is already complete at the time of purchase (Zemke & Schaaf, 1989, pp. 13–36).

A final but significant barrier to achieving satisfaction is the overvaluation of technology as the predominant solution to health care problems. This attitude must be balanced by a heartfelt belief in the healing nature of the nurse-patient relationship. If organizations acknowledge the power of this relationship, those individual attentions (long remembered by patients and families) become everyday occurrences on the nursing unit. Without such a focus at this level, attempts to achieve excellence, from the patient's viewpoint, will remain superficial.

Principles 3 and 4: Autonomy and Entrepreneurship, and Productivity through People

Principles 3 and 4 share a common theme related to beliefs about nursing staff and their work. Nursing staff beliefs include the following: (1) Nurses are good and trustworthy, (2) nurses are unique and should be treated as individuals, (3) nurses expect partnership and respect, (4) nurses do not dislike work, (5) nurses commit themselves to the extent that their own needs are met, and (6) nurses are self-managing (Porter O'Grady, 1986, pp. 25–42; Wowk, 1989, pp. 22–24). Traditional nursing management structures, however, are not grounded in these beliefs and thus produce relationships that are detached and impersonal. The new management challenge predominant in the excellence literature is not to tap physical resources in the worker, but rather his or her knowledge, spirituality, and emotions. The development of a people-valuing culture within an organization creates an intimacy that stimulates individuals to higher levels of productivity. What is significant about this management approach is that it is a "shift from command to consensus" (Miller, 1984, p. 40). This shift implies engaging the worker at both a personal and a professional level, stimulating excellence and innovation through participation.

Professional nurses who expect respect and partnership in their work settings will purposefully search for opportunities to be involved and to obtain any information necessary to do their work well. The presence of professional relationships creates an environment of trust in an organization, which in turn directly relates to the degree of nurses' commitment to excellence in practice (Porter O'Grady, 1986, pp. 25–42). The development of such partnerships in health care organizations is no easy feat. Power struggles, political history, information management issues, and time demands are all factors that must be addressed in order for partnerships to be successful. In the long run, however, such collaboration will move an organization to even higher levels of quality patient care.

The features of collaboration, communication, and individual recognition are strongly evident in magnet hospitals. Staff nurses have the support to use their own initiative to solve problems or implement innovation and to re-examine policies and procedures for effectiveness. Strong recognition and reward programs are tied to quality patient care (Kramer & Schmolenberg, 1988a, pp. 11–13).

Principle 5: Hands-On, Value-Driven Leadership

Unfortunately, many health care organizations still see their professional staff as providers rather than as partners in the patient care process. This perception conflicts with Peters and Waterman's descriptions of the nature of leader-subordinate relationships in excellent companies. Leadership in excellent companies can best be described as transformational. Such leaders are charismatic and instrumental in creating a collective vision, inspiring others to have the same degree of commitment. Transformational leaders engage in intense relationships with their subordinates, who in turn become leaders themselves. The values and the vision of the leader permeate all parts of the organization (Bennis & Nanus, 1985; Singer,

1985, pp. 143–146). In magnet hospitals, transformational leaders were evident in the nursing departments studied by Kramer and Schmolenberg (1988b, p. 13). The directors of nursing were described as charismatic, inspiring, and able to stir emotion. They often held national reputations and led well-educated and empowered teams of managers.

Principle 6: Stick to the Knitting

This principle of excellence refers to the ability to remain focused on the business central to an organization's mission—to do what the organization does best (Peters & Waterman, 1982, p. 293). Some diversification is all right, but too much will lead to failure. For example, some hospitals have tried to develop businesses that were not central to the issue of acute care services. Often such ventures failed because of inexperience with the for-profit sector and lack of knowledge about the product (Herzlinger, 1989, pp. 95–103).

In a similar vein, Jackson (1989, pp. 4–5) warned against the dire consequences of nursing not sticking to its knitting by taking on the responsibilities of other departments, particularly outside of the 7:00 A.M. to 4:00 P.M. business hours. The cutbacks in support services and the shifting of the eliminated services' tasks onto nursing is draining our nurses and threatening the quality of patient care. Delivery systems and resultant work expectations should be designed so that nurse and patient characteristics match, and so that nurses are not overloaded with the work of other departments.

Principle 7: Simple Form, Lean Management

This principle refers to the degree of complexity in an organizational structure. Complexity in health care organizations has resulted in segmented, highly specialized departments that do not communicate with one another. Decision making is slow because it has to move through tortuous layers of management review (Mintzberg, 1979). In excellent organizations, the structure is modified to enhance service. Magnet hospitals have several indicators of this principle present in their nursing departments. The traditional nursing supervisor role has been eliminated, and head nurses' span of control has been expanded to department head levels (Kramer & Schmolenberg, 1988b, p. 14).

Principle 8: Simultaneous Loose and Tight Properties

This principle refers to the ability of an organization to become more effective through centralization, while allowing for flexible structures that enhance collaboration. Moss Kanter (1989, pp. 55–90) observes that both centralized and decentralized organizations have problems that limit the achievement of excellence. Traditional centralized structures impede progress through cumbersome communication processes, power struggles, and support for the status quo. On the other hand, highly decentralized organizations are at times poorly coordinated and undisciplined. These limitations can be modified by centralizing those functions that will benefit from stability and decentralizing those functions that are obstructed by control. Interestingly, magnet hospitals display this characteristic, often centralizing documentation and policy and procedure while decentralizing problem-solving activities (Kramer & Schmolenberg, 1988b, pp. 13–14).

CULTURE BUILDING FOR EXCELLENCE

If the eight principles of excellence are woven into the very fabric of a nursing organization, a strong culture of excellence will prevail. This culture is reflected in the symbolic meanings assigned to members through their social surroundings and those meanings reinforced for newcomers or for those who stray from the fold (del Bueno & Freund, 1986, pp. 3–27).

What is a culture of excellence? It is one that encourages the integration of nurses' needs and hospital goals, stimulates dissatisfaction with the status quo, supports consensus decision making, rewards performance, values knowledge and learning, and promotes both integrity and intimacy in the provision of services to the patient.

Before discussing steps in the development of a culture of excellence, it is important to consider a potential threat to productivity that may arise during the process. This threat is what Curtain (1989, pp. 7–8) has referred to as the "performance edge." Leaders can set high goals and stimulate productivity, but the intensity of the work may in fact temporarily decrease rather than increase. Too much intensity drives nurses hard and threatens innovation because nurses are too tired to be creative. Therefore, it is imperative that a well-defined plan be developed, emphasizing strategies for the preparation of people for change as well as the implementation steps. The initial step for any plan is to assess the current status of the organization, so that a starting point for the change process can be identified. Can nurses at all levels and across the organization describe the mission and philosophy of the organization? Do they believe it? Do nurses see that their activities contribute to the mission? How are nursing leaders described? These and other questions will provide information as to any features of excellence that may already be predominant. The checklist in Appendix 2-A may be used to guide such an assessment.

After assessment is complete, nursing leaders can target elements and functions that require modification in order for excellence in the organization to be achieved.

A vision and a definition of excellence will be developed, reflecting the collective vision of all groups within the organization (Bennis & Nanus, 1985, pp. 184–214). This collective vision must be developed from the bottom up. It is here that the leader's role is key. Development of the vision must be directed as a collaborative process and yet be strongly influenced by the nursing leader's values. In addition, the leader will need to actively seek opportunities to articulate and reinforce the vision in a way that builds support across the organization.

However, reward systems and a collective vision are not enough to achieve excellence in patient care. Quality, as an indicator of excellence, must be defined. In the determination of quality, the standards, indicators, criteria, and outcomes must be established for specific customer groups. Interviews, focal groups, review of professional standards, complaint analysis, patient visits, hotlines, and patient advisory committees are useful approaches to the definition of quality. Furthermore, potential threats to quality patient care must be identified and pursued.

The vision and definition of quality will simply become lip service if rewards systems are not examined in relationship to the definitions and principles of excellence. Four basic areas must be examined: (1) Career ladders must reflect standards of excellence, (2) both career ladder opportunities and annual appraisals must be driven from the same set of performance standards, (3) hiring practices should reflect the identification of behaviors that support the achievement of excellence, and (4) nurses who do not meet standards should be quickly identified and provided opportunities to change, or be terminated.

Once quality has been defined, a service strategy must be delineated by the leadership group. This strategy will direct how and what resources will be applied to maximize opportunities and minimize threats to the achievement of excellence. Such a strategy can be developed for a specialty service such as orthopaedics, for a hospital department such as nursing or radiology, or for an entire organization. Regardless of its scope, a service strategy should be evaluated at least annually; standards of care and missions may change due to shifts in technology or changes in the resources available to provide the service. The three key elements of a service strategy are described below.

1. Statement of intent: This section summarizes the services to be provided, emphasizing standards of care and expected outcomes. The narrative links the new or modified service to the mission and philosophy of the organization and forms the basis for QA activities.
2. Marketing issues: Consumer satisfaction data and the opportunities for growth derived from these data are described in this section of the service strategy. The QA coordinator and the marketing department may pool some of their information in order to effectively analyze the market plan. Does the patient service have value in identified customer's eyes? Does the service

noticeably differentiate you from competitors? Is the service deliverable? Can it be offered in multiple sites?

3. Resource needs: This section addresses the knowledge, personnel, and material resources needed to achieve the strategy outlined (Zemke & Schaaf, 1989, pp. 37–46). A summary of the resources currently available to implement the strategy, along with the delineation of additional resource demands, is included in this section. Also, the fiscal impact of resource demands must be described so that the strategy can be evaluated from a cost perspective. What will fund the strategy? Will meeting the service strategy be a revenue opportunity? Will there be a start-up expense and then a point in time when revenue will begin to accrue to offset expenses?

The best service strategy will fail if it does not fit the culture, and the strongest culture will not overcome a poor strategy (Hickman & Silva, 1984, pp. 79–85). Consequently, an important step in the process of achieving excellence is to clearly evaluate the relationship of organizational culture and strategy. Commitment to a new service strategy must somehow match a nursing organization's traditional way of satisfying patient care needs. If an organization sees itself as a high-technology tertiary care center, then service strategies that focus on wellness or health promotion will be seen as peripheral to the main business and will fail due to lack of support.

For example, some contemporary hospitals have identified managed care programs (and their reviewers) as customers. Unfortunately, some nurses and physicians see managed care program requirements as burdensome and not in the best interest of patients. Managed care requirements may prohibit the provision of services the caregiver sees as necessary or may require a discharge date that seems premature to caregivers. Therefore, the interactions between reviewers and professionals can be strained and conflict-ridden. A service strategy to keep current managed care customers and gain new ones may fail because of lack of a good fit with the culture, or a lack of a plan to work with the incongruence.

SKILLS FOR THE PRACTITIONER OF EXCELLENCE

The attainment of excellence is a purposeful and developmental process, carefully crafted by a skilled nursing leader. The individual interested in building and maintaining a culture of excellence will engage in several key activities: planning and evaluation, skillful use of self, inspiring communications, consistency and presence, tolerance for honest mistakes, and empowerment through participation.

Careful planning provides not only direction but also benchmarks for the achievement of sometimes very abstract goals. A strategic plan is also a communication tool that can be used to prepare the organization and to keep nurses informed about progress on objectives. Re-education strategies, discussion groups, and incentive programs need to be tied to each objective so that the service strategy is equally understood across the organization. This leads to ongoing commitment and the development of reward systems that work for and not against the strategy.

The skillful use of self is central to effective leadership. This skill is the ability to always treat others with courtesy, to listen carefully to employee needs, and to treat each individual as an individual. It involves assuming a nonjudgmental stance, in which the manager of excellence accepts people for who they are while looking for opportunities to tie individual needs to organizational goals (Bennis & Nanus, 1985, pp. 184–214).

In order to develop a culture of excellence, the nursing leader must also be able to communicate a vision, which must remain firm even when the going gets rough (Bennis & Nanus, 1985, pp. 184–214). The consistency and predictability of a message inspires trust. Using key phrases and seeking opportunities to formally and informally communicate the vision are important communication approaches. In addition, the development of a strong group of supporters across the organization who can also carry the message will promote the development of trust. Thus people will be motivated to commit their energies to the vision.

Nursing leaders must be visible in the midst of change. In health care alone, the amount of change taking place is draining energy, stifling risk taking, and limiting creativity. Presence implies persistence, strength, and constancy of thought. In addition, the leader can assess the level of commitment as well as the degree to which the vision still matches the direction of an organization. A mismatch of organizational mission and service strategy for excellence portends failure and creates significant discomfort for those committed to the strategy.

The leader of an excellent organization must be comfortable with risk taking and tolerate errors. Failures must be redefined as opportunities for learning. This will take considerable work, since achieving success and avoiding failure is so ingrained in American culture. In the patient care arena, tolerance for mistakes is problematic, since errors can negatively influence patient outcomes. The assessment of what kinds of errors will be tolerated as opportunities for learning must be carefully communicated across the organization. QA findings can be used to identify skills or knowledge needed to reduce errors.

Finally, the practitioner of excellence empowers the providers of service through participation. A successful leader creates a community, a unity of purpose, through the integration of personal and organizational goals. As the achievement of these goals becomes evident, nurses recognize that they played a role in making something happen and that they could do it in the future. This is empowerment (Miller, 1984, pp. 67–84).

SUMMARY

Today's contemporary health care environment is extremely stressful. Scarce resources, very complex patient care demands, job security fears, and competition for market share combine to create an environment fraught with contradictions. It is an environment experienced with intensity. The notion of developing a culture of excellence in such a nursing environment is not an impossible dream. In fact, it may be the very salve that is needed to help nursing survive and thrive. The interpersonal relationships required for its successful implementation may help to reduce stress by limiting the isolation that often occurs in chaotic environments. A vision and standards for nursing excellence will instill hope in the future. The commitment to such a vision and the experience of being rewarded for excellence will allow us to reach into our reservoirs of energy and summon the strength we need to continue to strive for quality patient care. Careful planning, recognition of the developmental nature of change, and balance in the process of change, so as not to intensify stress, are the guideposts to success. As professional nurses, we made a commitment to serve. We cannot let this opportunity to improve the quality of care escape from us, simply because these are chaotic times.

REFERENCES

Bennis, W., & Nanus, B. (1985). *Leaders*. New York: Harper & Row.

Cleverley, W.O., & Stetson, R.L. (1985). In search of excellence: Fact or fiction? *Hospital and Health Services Administration, 30*, 26–47.

Curtain, L. (1989). The performance edge. *Nursing Management, 20*, 7–8.

del Bueno, D.J., & Freund, C. (1986). *Power and policies in nursing administration*. Owings Mills, MD: Rynd.

Herzlinger, R.E. (1989). The failed revolution in health care. *Harvard Business Review, 67*, 95–103.

Hickman, C.R., & Silva, M.A. (1984). *Creating excellence*. New York: New American Library.

Jackson, B. (1989). Ownership imbalance. *Journal of Nursing Administration, 9*, 4–5.

Kramer, M., & Schmolenberg, C. (1988a). Magnet hospitals: 1. Institutions of excellence. *Journal of Nursing Administration, 18*, 13–24.

Kramer, M., & Schmolenberg, C. (1988b). Magnet hospitals: 2. Institutions of excellence. *Journal of Nursing Administration, 18*, 11–19.

Lynn, M. (1990, February). *Quality of nursing care: A new beginning*. Paper presented at Sigma Theta Tau's Research Day (Beta Upsilon chapter), Phoenix, AZ.

Miller, L.M. (1984). *American spirit: Visions of a new corporate structure*. New York: Warner Books.

Mintzberg, H. (1979). *The Structuring of Organizations*. New York: Prentice-Hall.

Moss Kanter, R. (1989). *When giants learn to dance*. New York: Simon & Schuster.

Naisbitt, J. (1984). *Megatrends*. New York: Warner Books.

Peters, T., & Austin, N. (1985). *A passion for excellence*. New York: Random House.

Peters, T., & Waterman, R.H., Jr. (1982). *In search of excellence*. New York: Harper & Row.

Porter O'Grady, T. (1986). *Creative nursing administration*. Gaithersburg, MD: Aspen Publishers.

Porter O'Grady, T., & Finnegan, S. (1984). *Shared governance for nursing.* Gaithersburg, MD: Aspen Publishers.

Singer, M.S. (1985). Transformation vs. transactional leadership: A study of New Zealand company managers. *Psychological Reports, 57,* 143–146.

Wowk, P. (1989). Partnering: A new strategy for nursing leadership. *Health Care Excellence, 32,* 22–24.

Zemke, R., & Schaaf, D. (1989). *The service edge.* New York: New American Library.

Assessing Your Department for Excellence

The following checklist can serve as a tool for developing preliminary strategies for enhancing excellence in patient care. Check the response that best describes your department.

1 = Never   4 = Usually
2 = Rarely   5 = Always
3 = Sometimes

	1	2	3	4	5
1. Bias for Action					
Multidisciplinary ad hoc task forces are commonly formed to solve problems.	—	—	—	—	—
Information about patient care issues is not limited to role or positions.	—	—	—	—	—
Nurses believe they are kept informed about patient care issues.	—	—	—	—	—
There is a positive, questioning attitude among the nursing staff.	—	—	—	—	—
Nurses have the authority to make certain patient care decisions.	—	—	—	—	—
There are collaborative structures in place, such as joint practice committees.	—	—	—	—	—
Unit-based quality assurance committees are empowered to initiate change.	—	—	—	—	—

	1	2	3	4	5

2. Customer Care

The patients cared for in your area can accurately describe your service.

The patient satisfaction tool is critically evaluated on a regular basis, and modifications are made based on the evaluation.

Nurses in your department intervene effectively with difficult patients and families.

Patient complaints, both written and verbal, are trended and shared with your department.

Nurses, physicians, and administrators agree upon the definition of the customer.

Quality assurance is a multidisciplinary function.

Your nursing department is recognized for an innovative program at the local, state, or national level.

3. People Orientation

The nursing staff exhibits a high degree of job satisfaction and commitment to the organization.

The professional disciplines who provide care trust one another and are proud to be associated with one another.

Nurse managers are viewed positively by their staff and by other department heads.

Nurses at the bedside have adequate opportunities to participate in patient care decision making at the unit and the nursing department levels.

Staff nurses can describe their work in relationship to the department's goals.

Staff nurses see themselves as full partners with other disciplines and with administrators in the delivery of patient care.

	1	2	3	4	5

4. Simultaneous Loose/Tight Properties

In your department, are the right services centralized for maximum efficiency?

Non-nursing, time-consuming functions are contracted to outside vendors.

All programs and services are well designed and controlled.

5. Culture of Excellence

Nurses perceive a personal benefit to belonging to your organization.

Reward systems reflect the standards of excellence.

Hiring practices result in a staff who can achieve excellence.

Nurses who cannot meet standards are dealt with in a timely and effective manner.

Quality is clearly defined and described as a value by the nursing staff.

6. Manager/Leader Self-Study

Planning and plan implementation are regular activities in your department.

As a leader, you make it your business to continually identify how you are seen and make changes as needed.

You accept people for who they are and for where they are in their own development.

You spend a consistent portion of your time in staff development.

You are a skilled public speaker.

Your words and your behavior match.

	1	2	3	4	5

You are comfortable with risks.

Those whom you work with know that you see mistakes as learning opportunities.

7. Leadership

Unit-based quality assurance activities produce information used in hospital strategic planning.

The nursing administration team is described by the professional nursing staff as leaders.

Staff nurses can accurately describe the director of nursing's value system.

The nursing director is visible and known to the staff.

8. Sticking to the Knitting

There is a clear distinction between nursing and non-nursing roles.

The nursing care assignments are planned in such a way to match patient needs with nursing skill.

Nurses are not asked to function in new roles without adequate development and assessment of their skills.

The nursing department has the necessary nursing expertise to provide new programs.

9. Simple Form/Lean Management

There is a reasonable manager to staff ratio.

Nursing staff feel that problems are addressed by administration in a timely and efficient manner.

Policies and procedures of the appropriate number and complexity are available to staff.

Directions for Scoring

99–0   You have a lot of work to do to develop a culture of excellence.

149–100   Some of the characteristics of excellence are present and can be a basis for growth.

199–150   Many of the characteristics of excellence are present. Some fine tuning is needed.

240–200   Your department is a model of excellence.

3

Cost and Quality: Are They Compatible?

Virginia Del Togno-Armanasco, MN, RN, Coordinator, Nursing Case Management, Tucson Medical Center, Tucson, Arizona

Susan Harter, MBA, RN, Director, Finance, Budget and Staffing, Tucson Medical Center, Tucson, Arizona

Nannette L. Goddard, MS, RN, Consultant and Lecturer, Specializing in Financial Planning and Management Systems for Nursing, Houston, Texas

One of the major challenges for nurse executives in today's health care environment is to balance the very real concerns about the costs of providing patient care with the need for assuring a quality product. In 1989 health care consumed over 11.5% of the gross national product (Kimball, 1990). With the expectation that costs will continue to rise, the federal government, health care providers, and employers are actively seeking ways to curtail these costs. Medical insurance premiums of corporations jumped 20%, and business paid more than one fifth of the total national health bill (Yeater, 1984). Medicare and Medicaid patients are responsible for 45% of the gross revenues in community hospitals (Gross, 1986). As a result, more pressure is being directed toward hospitals to identify the costs of care and to deliver care in a more efficient and effective manner, while maintaining quality. Since the payroll for nursing department employees comprises 50% or more of the entire wage and salary expense in most hospitals, it becomes obvious that this pressure will be passed along to nurse executives, nurse managers, and nursing staff.

Bedside nurses tell anyone who will listen that no more money can be saved at the bedside without affecting the quality of care patients receive. They are experiencing the pressures of "downsizing," cost containment, and overall decreased staffing. In many instances the identification of what work needs to be done, by whom, and when, in order for the patient and all caregivers to feel the satisfaction and benefits of quality interventions and outcomes, has not been made. The challenge is how to deliver the best care for the lowest possible cost. As a result, measuring productivity becomes paramount to ensure that we are spending our health care dollars appropriately to deliver a quality product.

The primary issue in addressing such a subject is that although costs can be identified in an objective manner, quality has been viewed as more subjective in nature. When nurses express a concern that they will be decreasing the quality of their care, they often have difficulty in expressing exactly which components of quality will be decreasing. This is not to negate their concerns, but rather to point out that the issue of quality in health care has been one of the "soft" parameters, and as such it is difficult to exactly measure or to even define. In many ways, quality is commonly held to be synonymous with excellence. Therefore, for quality to be defined in a meaningful manner, structure, process, and outcomes must first be defined and identified for nursing practice standards (Krueger Wilson, 1986). These standards must be based on accepted measures of excellence in nursing care delivery. However, each illness is unique, and each professional who decides the services needed for its treatment uses a distinct judgment process that is also unique. Thus the problem of defining quality is a many-faceted challenge.

Costs, on the other hand, are more objective. They include *direct care costs*, in terms of hours and total related salaries; *indirect care costs*, including management time and nonproductive time such as sick, vacation, holiday, and education time; and *administrative costs* or "institutional overhead," covering plant operations, maintenance, depreciation, and nonpatient charge departments such as laundry, transportation, risk management, security, and the like.

ISSUES IN PATIENT CARE DELIVERY

Since neither cost nor quality alone address the real health services issues pertaining to the two items combined, it becomes essential that the coordination and integration of both must be assessed, in terms of the elements addressed by the following questions (VanderVeen, 1988):

1. If the job was done right, was it done on time?
2. If it was done right and on time, was it cost-effective?
3. If it was right, on time, and cost-effective, were the desired outcomes achieved?
4. Is there another outcome that could be a quality outcome for this patient?

Thus cost and quality must be valued equally. Resources must be dedicated to identifying both the cost of providing patient care and the quality standards to establish for each patient, based on the structure, process, and outcomes of the care delivery process. However, this is not a simple process, as reliability and validity measures of quality in nursing are missing. This is compounded by the fact that clinical practice and its delivery processes vary according to the organizational environment in which the care is delivered. This environment affects nurses, patients, and others in health care settings. The environment includes the hospital characteristics and culture, patient unit organization, social-physiological variables among the staff, leadership characteristics, and nursing education, as well as the availability of housekeeping, administrative, and clerical services (Hegyvary, 1988).

Evaluating Productivity

In order to achieve some sense of relationship between cost and quality, the productiveness of the workers and the system must be examined. How well are resources used in producing output (patient care)? How much does it cost to produce one unit of output (a patient day)?

Productivity is the relationship between output produced and the input required to achieve that output. Productivity is usually expressed as a percentage describing the ratio between units of output to units of input.

$$\text{Productivity} \ = \ \frac{\text{Output}}{\text{Input}} \ = \ \frac{\text{Results}}{\text{Costs}}$$

Productivity also implies some standard of what ought to be and should be examined as trends over a period of time (Spitzer & Priselac, 1986, pp. 7–8).

Let us examine the two components of the equation. An unweighted unit of service (UOS) is the most basic *output*. In nursing that would be the patient day. However, a more accurate measure of output must factor in intensity; thus the patient day would be acuity adjusted.

$$\text{Output} = \text{Patient day} \times \text{acuity factor}$$

("Acuity factor" is the weighted UOS.)

Input can be measured in a number of ways. Productive time, worked hours, or paid hours are all methods of measuring input. It is valuable to track information using more than one method. Worked hours per weighted UOS can assist the manager in evaluating how productively the staff performs. The problem with this definition of productivity is that it considers only the cost of direct nursing care and ignores indirect nursing care and ancillary and overhead costs. By tracking paid hours per weighted UOS, the manager can evaluate how well sick, vacation, holiday, and, in some instances, education time is being planned and used across the months.

$$\text{Input} \ = \ \text{Worked hours}$$
$$\text{or}$$
$$\text{Input} \ = \ \text{Paid hours}$$

$$\frac{\text{Output}}{\text{Input}} = \frac{\text{Weighted UOS}}{\text{Worked hours or worked hours per weighted UOS}}$$

$$\frac{\text{Output}}{\text{Input}} = \frac{\text{Weighted UOS}}{\text{Paid hours or paid hours per weighted UOS}}$$

There are a number of different patient classification or acuity systems; however, their purposes are the same. By either identifying nursing tasks or patient needs, the caregiver can quickly identify and quantify necessary nursing care for an individual patient. The patient classification system then groups patients to identify required staffing for a given nursing unit. Some systems also group patients in a manner that allows comparisons of resource use across nursing units. Patient classification systems are useful productivity measurement tools because they reflect nursing's involvement with patients, as opposed to the way nursing fits into the medical model of care. In addition, they are designed to provide information regarding patient needs on a daily basis, and monitoring the system's data can be readily accomplished.

Some systems utilize patient care activities as proxy measures for health outcomes (i.e., hospital patient days) (Helt & Jelinek, 1988). Another system, based on the postulate that *severity of illness* and *quality of care* are related (Panniers, 1987), classifies patients in terms of age, body system involved in the illness, stage of the disease, complications, and the patient's response to the therapy. Chronic diseases such as diabetes or pulmonary disease, age, location of pathology, and iatrogenic factors impact resource use as measured by any system.

Given all these factors, Donabedian (1984) notes that quality of health care depends on choosing the appropriate objectives of care and selecting appropriate ways to attain them. Depending upon the objective (i.e., health or a movement toward wellness), the areas of responsibility of the health care professionals must be determined. Through a joint decision made by both the health care practitioner and a fully informed client, decisions can be made that are both feasible and desired. This strategy has two major components, one technical and one interpersonal. Both must be implemented jointly by the client and practitioner for success to be achieved.

Concern about the methods to obtain the objectives of care is a change of focus on the part of health care professionals. This change of focus has highlighted the inadequacies of some of the more common definitions of nursing productivity. For example, output is often stated in terms of quantity of services rendered. As of yet, it is not possible to define output in terms of value of services rendered. Inasmuch as caring is the chief ingredient that goes into the process of delivering care, it is not completely clear what constitutes the "quality" of service, as this output is not easily distinguishable from the input of the system (Omachonu & Nanda, 1989).

Another definition of productivity *compares actual nursing care hours to required nursing care hours*. However, this is a definition of efficiency rather than productivity, as efficiency is the ratio of actual output attained to the standard output expected. A second problem with this definition is that it implies that productivity can be increased by reducing the required nursing care hours or by increasing the number of actual nursing care hours.

Multiple factors in the nursing care arena can promote or adversely affect productivity. These include patients' condition or acuity, staffing considerations, physician-nurse inter-relationships, availability of technological advances, amount of computerization in use, ancillary services, and hospital characteristics (i.e., physician environment, culture, and the availability of health care alternatives) (Hoffman, 1988, pp. 60–61). Few of these areas can be measured objectively. Patient classification and related staffing are exceptions, and the most manageable way to consistently measure nursing productivity. These measurements can also be used to identify the cost of the services rendered and the resources expended.

True productivity measures must eventually consider the results of nursing interventions, the ability to restore good health to a patient or enhance a peaceful death (Omachonu & Nanda, 1989). Although difficult to measure, these quality issues are ultimately the most important focus for most nurses in health care settings.

EVALUATING QUALITY IN HEALTH CARE

Process

To evaluate quality, each health care facility must first define and accept for itself a concept of quality. Secondly, it must identify all cost factors affecting the achievement of this quality. Once these concepts are defined and identified, they must be integrated into the facility's daily operational components. These actions result in the identification of patient care service as an essential indicator of the organization's overall performance (Fralic, 1988).

Examples of *quality indicators* that can be utilized are the achievement level of nursing care standards, length of stay variances attributable to nursing actions, infection rates, and patient incidents attributable to nursing action. *Cost indicators* affecting the achievement of quality that need to be evaluated are compliance-to-staffing standards, professional-to-nonprofessional personnel ratios, budgeted-to-filled positions, patient acuity, and compliance to salary and non-salary budgets (Fralic, 1988).

In the absence of clearly defined quality and cost outcome goals, confusion occurs among the institution's major players regarding the agreement, coordination, and achievement of such goals. As a result, inappropriate action choices are implemented, resulting in a less acceptable standard of care and a "climate of negligence" (Currie, 1987). Interdepartmental controversies and communication and coordination problems contribute to the confusion. Thus quality care standards and goals must be specific to the problem being addressed (Everett, 1985).

Challenge

Providing quality patient care within a cost-restrictive reimbursement system is a major concern of health care professionals in today's changing health care environment. This is well documented in the literature by surveys of both physicians and nurses.

In a survey of physicians regarding their perception of how cost restrictions were affecting patient care, two thirds responded that patients were being injured by cost control measures such as the prospective payment system. They stated that "we are being forced to cheat the system in order to provide the patient with the care we are trained to give" (Crane, 1986).

Critical care nurses surveyed identified 11 negative effects of cost-cutting measures on the quality of care being provided to patients in critical care units (Grif Alspach, 1986):

1. increased patient-nurse ratios
2. premature patient discharge
3. increased use of float, temporary, and nursing aide staff
4. little time available for patient education, discharge care planning, or continuity of care
5. readmission of patients shortly after transfer from critical care units
6. increased patient acuity
7. receiving units unable to provide necessary care
8. greater number of procedures ordered to offset the diagnosis-related group (DRG) reimbursement system
9. larger medical centers refusing to accept patients who lack health insurance coverage
10. less attention paid by physicians to patients who lack ability to pay health care costs
11. reversion to team nursing

Interestingly, these same nurses identified 5 positive effects of cost-cutting measures on quality of care (Grif Alspach, 1986):

1. more efficient use of critical care beds and services
2. more complete documentation
3. greater awareness of patient needs for care
4. retention of only the better nurses
5. more aggressive medical treatment

Criteria for Solution

In 1986 a panel of experts composed of physicians, government policy makers, and an attorney identified the criteria to be addressed in determining if the cost containment methodologies currently in place were affecting quality of care (O'Donnell, Griffith, Donnell, Fuchs, Jencks, Doan, & Nestler, 1986):

1. Are there premature discharges of patients, with no place for many of them to go?
2. Are there increased numbers of adverse consequences (i.e., death, disability, pain, and suffering)?

These criteria must be included in quality assurance (QA) programs in order to ascertain if quality outcomes are being achieved in a cost containment environment.

To determine if discharged patients are ready and able to assume the care needed for their continued recuperation at home, all members of the health care team must participate in prospective planning. They must determine the organizational supports required to provide patient care that meets established standards and requirements (Beyers, 1986). These actions can be facilitated by key individuals in the organization working together to establish efficient and effective management practices needed for efficient and effective clinical practices.

Persons and practices are interdependent in providing patient care and cannot be separated. Thus organizational inputs affecting the quality of care must be systematically monitored and constantly corrected to promote the delivery of planned care. It again reinforces the need for nursing to respond to these changes and incorporate not only productivity based on hours worked according to patient classification but also nursing practice patterns based on nursing standards, nursing diagnosis, and nursing process. In other words, how the nurse spends his or her time, rather than how much time is spent, is the criterion that most affects the balancing of cost and quality (Beyers, 1986).

Results

As stated earlier, quality health care in today's health care environment depends on a choice of appropriate objectives of care and appropriate ways to attain them. Each individual patient in any specific situation and the health care practitioners responsible for the patient's care must be fully informed in order to participate in joint decisions as to what amount of improvement, in what aspects of health, are both feasible and desired. With this approach, quality monitoring, followed by corrective action, can reduce the cost of care by eliminating useless or potentially harmful care. However, it must be acknowledged that quality monitoring followed by corrective action can also *add* to the cost of care by helping to correct the discrepancy between current performance and the higher level of quality to which all involved aspire. When monetary cost enters the definition of quality, there is a trade-off between cost and improvements in health (Donabedian, 1984).

Consumer Satisfaction

The current trend in the health care community is to make quality the top priority as a differentiation strategy positioning institutions for a competitive advantage. However, for it to be effective, "high quality" must *first* be defined by the customers, not the providers. Therefore, each health care facility or provider must identify these important "customers" and their criteria for quality in order to assure success in this area. Some examples of the typical customers of health care facilities are patients, physicians, and employees/nursing staff. These customers must define the value of "quality" from the perspective of what service or services are deemed high quality at the right price.

Integration of the customer's identified quality components into the organization must be accomplished through departmental standards and policies that reflect these values. Measurement must be conducted throughout the process, and performance adjusted as necessary, based upon feedback from the market. Additionally, these actions must be communicated to the customers in a format they understand and accept (Jensen, 1988). In the hospital or health care environment, such service quality is determined through the human performance of the hospital staff. As a result, hospitals and other health care organizations must incorporate the assurance of quality inside their organizations and not look to inspectors for regulation from the outside.

Outcome Measures in Health Care

To achieve a quality product, Lewis, Nitta, Biczi, and Robinson (1986, p. 19) list 10 critical factors or outcome-related measures:

1. *Communication:* gives accurate verbal shift-to-shift report.
2. *Guest Relations:* communicates effectively and establishes good relationships with other disciplines.
3. *Problem-Oriented Medical Charting:* identifies and knows current condition as well as changes in the past 24 hours of all assigned patients and can report care plans for each.
4. *Care Planning:* establishes nursing care goals within the framework of the medical care plan.
5. *Medication Therapy:* meets standards of practice related to medication administration.

6. *Infection Control Techniques:* meets standards of practice related to infection control.
7. *IV Therapy:* meets standards of practice of intravenous therapy.
8. *Patient Hygiene:* coordinates patients' daily hygienic needs for cleanliness and acceptable appearance.
9. *Response to Care:* creates an atmosphere of mutual trust, acceptance, and respect.
10. *Patient Education and Discharge Planning:* utilizes available resources related to discharge planning.

Some or all of these must be considered and/or incorporated in measuring the achievement of quality, cost-effective patient care.

Difficulty in Isolating Variables

Given the ability to identify appropriate outcome measures in health care, variables that are components of these outcome measures or standards of care must be isolated, which is a difficult matter. One reason for this difficulty is the unique nature of each illness and the elusive factor of professional judgment required to decide what services are needed (Gross, 1986). Cost assumptions must include the nursing department's obligation to measure actual patient care cost against the quality outcome expectation. This requires a major shift in the way standards are defined. Using this perspective, planned, required, and actually delivered care must be compared and evaluated.

The Joint Commission on Accreditation of Healthcare Organizations, in an effort to encourage health care facilities to identify and utilize these variables, or standards of care, recommends that 1% of hospital costs be expended on QA activities. Some of the activities they identify as essential are the monitoring and evaluation of all major aspects of care, resolving important problems and taking opportunities to improve patient care, developing criteria, and evaluating the effectiveness of the program (Syron & Corey, 1989).

A second national group that is attempting to assist nursing departments to identify features of high-quality, cost-effective nursing care is the National Commission of Nursing Implementation Project, Features of High-Quality, Cost-Effective Nursing Care Delivery Systems of the Future (National Commission on Nursing Implementation Project, 1988, pp. 1–6). This group has identified four major characteristics of effective, high-quality, cost-effective nursing departments: delivery-related features, evaluation-related features, market-related features, and policy-related features.

Included among the *delivery-related features* are (1) working relationships among nurses, physicians, and other members of the health care team; (2) roles that incorporate authority, autonomy, and responsibility and offer appropriate compensation; (3) involvement of nurse managers in preparing the budget, managing resource utilization, and preserving a safe practice climate with acceptable outcomes; and (4) market knowledge concerning the ability to efficiently produce a service that will sell or draw consumers.

Evaluation-related features include (1) mechanisms for determining consumer satisfaction and providing feedback to the unit and to the practitioner, along with the monitoring of retention rates; (2) a consumer feedback mechanism; (3) supervisor and peer evaluation; and (4) a nursing QA program. Additional components of this criterion are (1) an evaluation mechanism for regarding cost-effectiveness, comparing standards and productivity standards; (2) a reliable and valid classification system; (3) information systems with outcome measures; (4) staff participation in designing cost accounting and reporting systems; and (5) staff education about the systems.

Market-related features include features that affect the demand for nursing services, such as (1) the involvement of practicing nurses in the selection and evaluation of technology and programming used in the provision of client care, (2) information systems that track utilization patterns, (3) consumer input and regular program evaluation, and (4) nurses' being involved in public relation activities of the organization.

The *policy-related features* identified affect nursing's ability to influence overall policies in the organization. These include (1) nursing's being formally placed to influence policy formation and implementation relevant to the organization as a whole, (2) nurses in middle management and clinical positions being members of institutional committees that set policy and procedure for patient care at the operational and patient unit levels, and (3) nursing's being positioned for accountability and authority over the fiscal resources for nursing practice.

EVALUATING COST IN HEALTH CARE

The cost for nursing services has two components. The first is the price to the environment, or that portion of the hospital's charges attributable to nursing services. This price is reflected on the bill to the patient or a third-party payer, usually as part of the room rate. The second price is the one that is internal to the institution. These are the resources allocated to the nursing department or a transfer price when nursing is charged to a product line. This is the "price" that is reflected in the budget (Skydell & Arndt, 1988). Three of the more common cost and work measurement systems used in nursing departments are (1) *patient classification systems*, which identify patients' needs more accurately and thus assign staff on the basis of patient need; (2) *relative value matrices*, used to determine the nursing care requirement associated with various high-volume diagnoses, surgical procedures, and DRGs; and (3) *split cost-accounting systems*, which have three components. The first is a *one-time fee*, charged to all patients for services such as admitting, billing, and medical records; the second is a *patient day fee*, charged for daily room and board in addition to other services typically associated with a hospital day, such as pharmaceutical and medical supplies; and the third is a *nursing care fee*, which represents the average nursing care requirements provided to patients according to illness and length of stay (Skydell & Arndt, 1988).

It has been postulated that in order to better control costs, consideration must be given to both the front room operations where the patient is present and the back room operations where the patient is absent. Additionally, the dual administrative structure—the supply side (constituting the hospital's administration, providing sufficient capacity of resources subsequently used) and the demand side (constituting the physician whose decisions result in resource utilization)—must be considered. This results in a cost control focus that includes a decrease in the cost of resources used (back room operations) and a decrease in the volume of resources used (front room operations). As a result, a system is provided that is flexible and designed to evolve and reduce undesired variability in the process (Rhea, 1986).

The dilemma of continuing to provide high-quality care in light of diminishing resources is one that strikes all medical staffs. Thus the use of an automated clinical/financial database in hospitals points the way to improvements in the cost and quality of health care. Utilization of services is largely under the control of physicians; therefore, efforts at diminishing utilization must focus upon them. Curtailing unnecessary utilization should decrease morbidity and mortality through elimination of the risks of unneeded diagnostic or therapeutic procedures, as well as via the reductions of errors in diagnosis resulting from unnecessary tests or procedures. However, if needed services are curtailed, the quality of care will be adversely affected. Thus opportunities for cost containment will be identified principally by comparison of actual practice patterns to expected practices (Mushlin, 1984).

Since excessive or unnecessary care implies poor quality of care and may also be harmful, QA strives to eliminate unnecessary services. The elusive balance that produces the optimal health result, and the indicators to measure that precise combination, demand our energetic scrutiny. Focusing on efficiency in implementing quality activities may lead us to define some key quality of care indicators, to streamline the implementation of care programs (Clemenhagen, 1987).

The success of any cost containment program depends on commitment of all the players to an accountable quality program. One way to achieve this commitment is to establish a goal and an accompanying plan for patient care as early as possible in the patient's disease process (VanderVeen, 1988). These objectives must be communicated to everyone on the clinical care team. The nurse's role in such a process is in serving as a facilitator to bring families and other clinical disciplines together in understanding and working together toward achieving the goals of the care process.

The "quick fix" of cutting costs is not the answer. It is predicted that up to 3000 hospitals will close their doors by 1992. The first to go will be those who have tried a "quick fix" and not defined their product accurately, or who have so diluted and adulterated their product that it is no longer worth its purchase price. Decisions about admission, discharge, referral, and even diversification into long-term and home health care can and should be based upon patient acuity rather than medical diagnosis alone. This reflects the fact that acuity increases as lengths of stay decrease, and as lengths of stay decrease, hospitals are downsizing. To maximize assets, hospitals must carefully combine *material resources* (technology, build-ings, grounds, equipment, and supplies), *capital* (money, bonds, investments, and credit), *labor* (nurses, physicians, technicians, support personnel), and *entrepreneurship* (the skill needed to blend the other three in the right quantity, at the right time, and in the right place to produce the right product). As a result, the immediate decisions about the deployment of resources, labor, and even capital equipment are enormously important (Curtin, 1986). The arena has shifted from a "treatment at any cost" environment to a competitive, cost-driven industry (Gillis, 1987). As a result, health care providers now must make decisions using the same criteria as other businesses.

Fuchs (1981) noted, "We do not, as the critics imply, have an option between evaluating and not evaluating. The only option is whether to evaluate explicitly, systematically, and openly, as cost benefit analysis/cost effectiveness analysis forces us to do, or whether to evaluate implicitly, haphazardly, and secretly, as has been done so often in the past." As a result, it is important to identify the differences between cost-benefit analysis and cost-effectiveness analysis. In cost-benefit analysis, a monetary value is assigned to all costs and benefits of a potential program, practice, or product. Thus the choice would be the lower cost-benefit ratio. In a cost-effectiveness analysis, a monetary value is not placed on benefits. However, all the costs, measured in dollars, necessary to achieve a certain effect (benefit) are calculated and expressed as cost/unit effectiveness (e.g., cost of vaccine program/amount of infectious disease prevented). This analysis is gener-ally used to compare the relative costs of several alternative programs, products, or practices that are designed to achieve the same objective.

Another way of examining this concept is by use of Williamson's definition of cost analysis. In it he defines *efficacy* as the ability of the intervention to produce the intended benefit to a defined population under ideal conditions, *effectiveness* as the extent of benefit achieved under usual condition, and *efficiency* as the extent to which benefit is achieved with a minimum of unnecessary expenditure of resources. The limitation of such cost analysis is that it is unable to measure some benefits such as pain and stress reduction, improved quality of life, or prevention of disability. It is also unable to measure some costs, such as education, transportation, premature debility or loss of life, or emotional distress. Such measures are based on a value judgment, subject to bias, personal opinion, and manipulation. Thus predicting future costs and benefits and discounting their present value is difficult. In conclusion, cost analysis itself is costly (Larson & Peters, 1986).

In light of all of the above information, it is obvious that nursing will play a critical role in the success or failure of hospital efforts to survive, since nursing occupies an essential position in the primary mission of hospitals, that of providing quality care to patients (Blaney, Hobson, & McHenry, 1988).

ETHICS, COST, AND QUALITY

The President's Commission for the Study of Ethical Problems in Medicine and Biomedical and Behavioral Research stated that society has an ethical obligation to ensure equitable access to health care for all. The commission further noted that efforts to contain rising health care costs are important but should not focus on limiting the attainment of equitable access for the least well served portion of the public. As a result of the implementation of the DRG prospective payment system, which attempts to control the inflationary cost of health care and to establish an average price system based on diagnosis, costs were reduced 10% to 40% (Crisham, 1986).

A recent panel of experts identified as a key concern the new emphasis on early discharge. It was perceived that for some patients there is no appropriate place for them to receive the follow-up care they required. They also noted that the effects of the three most adverse consequences, death, disability, and pain and suffering, had not yet been calculated (Crisham, 1986).

These concerns have placed nursing in several moral dilemmas regarding (1) the patient's right to know and right to have meaningful involvement in health care decisions, (2) the promotion and definition of quality of life, (3) the maintenance of professional and institutional standards, and (4) the distribution of nursing resources.

A recent study of nurses regarding how cost containment activities were affecting their practice noted that they perceived cost containment as hurting the quality of care. They stated that they have "no time for a caring attitude" and that a much higher value is placed on counting statistics than on comforting. As a result, caring is the first thing to go. They further note that patient assessments are made "on the run," resulting in care that is not always safe (Collins, 1988).

Physicians are also concerned with the pressure that is being placed on them to reduce costs. Their premise is that providing care and attempting to control costs must not occur at the expense of the patient's life or safety, or compromise the quality of care being provided. They do acknowledge that they must be active partners in cooperative arrangements to reduce the duplication of expensive services. They also acknowledge that they must be willing to be innovative in providing alternative means of care (Gordinier, 1985).

Another factor that health care practitioners must incorporate into their assessment of the cost-quality dilemma is their obligation to provide the most effective care efficiently. However, when added benefits are small relative to added cost, practitioners may stop short of the most effective care, in obedience to patient preferences. As health care becomes more highly organized and more fully financed under public or quasi-public auspices, health care practitioners will be called upon to serve in the capacity of judges, arbiters, and rationers. Thus they are poised at a crossroads in the health care delivery system (Donabedian, 1988).

NEWER MODELS OF NURSING CARE DELIVERY

Since preferred provider organizations and prospective payment systems have shifted some of the responsibility for controlling costs to health care providers, it becomes mandatory that health care providers become knowledgeable about available options. One such option is case management. It is presented as a tool for improving patient care through the coordination of health care services, to ensure that patients receive appropriate and high-quality care (Fisher, 1987). As a result, the decade of the 1980s saw the development of many case management models. Each model attempts to unite the concepts of patient care organization and quality within an efficient and effective patient care delivery environment. Examples are the differentiated practice model, managed care/case management, professional practice/case management, and collaborative nursing case management.

Differentiated Practice Model

Differentiated practice as developed by the National Commission on Nursing Implementation Project under the leadership of Dr. Primm is a care delivery system that combines the model of primary nursing for all clients with a case management model for the chronically ill or for those with no support system in the home. Its goal is to place nursing in a strategic position to influence hospital operations and medical practice. Some of the potential benefits of differentiated nursing practice include effective deployment of nursing staff into emerging new roles, shared governance that facilitates staff nurse involvement in the clinical decision-making process, and increased clinical management skills, resulting in integration and continuity of care and substantial cost savings (National Commission on Nursing Implementation Project, 1988).

Managed Care/Case Management

Managed care/case management as developed at New England Medical Center, Boston, Massachusetts, is described as both a model and a technology for restructuring the clinical production process and roles that facilitate beneficial cost-quality outcomes. It is a proactive response by nursing to restructure the tools and roles to better fit the demands of today's environment.

To ensure positive cost-quality outcomes, the case manager in this model is a central caregiver to the patients in his or her caseload. This nurse is responsible for the patient's entire episode of care, as well as for developing formal collaborative practice groups. It is a new way of planning, managing, and thinking about nursing's role in health care delivery (Zander, 1988).

Professional Practice/Case Management

Professional practice/case management as practiced at St. Mary's Hospital, Tucson, Arizona, is another attempt to integrate cost control with quality in health care. Through an emphasis on pre- and posthospital care, this model attempts to integrate all of the nursing care needed by the client through a nursing network. The nursing network seeks to strengthen nurses as professionals and enable them to contribute the full range of their expertise in promoting health. Within the nursing network, professional nurse case managers are accountable for the quality and cost-effectiveness of nursing care, as well as for promoting access to health care for individuals. Professional nurse case management is credited with helping to turn many of the hospital's unprofitable service areas into profit makers (Ethridge, 1989).

Collaborative Nursing Case Management

Collaborative nursing case management, as developed at Tucson Medical Center, Tucson, Arizona, is a formalized multidisciplinary and integrated process for planning and delivering continuity of care for the purpose of achieving a balance among appropriate patient outcomes, efficiency, quality, and cost-effectiveness. Some of the goals of this program are to promote collaborative practice, coordination of care, and continuity of care among physicians, nurses, and ancillary departments; to facilitate the achievement of expected and/or standardized patient outcomes with an individual, human touch; and to promote appropriate reduced utilization of resources. Using a research protocol, early results demonstrate that resource utilization is improved, and patient, physician, and nurse satisfaction is enhanced (Del Togno-Armanasco, Olivas, & Harter, 1989).

Case Management by Health Care Payers

Another type of case management utilized by health care payers focuses on the less than 1% of its clients who incur between 25% and 50% of a plan's expenditures. It attempts to coordinate and utilize health care resources appropriately in a quality and cost-effective manner (Kenkel, 1985). Case managers are charged with identifying high-risk patients and arranging for the provision of health care for these patients in the most cost-effective setting. Case management is not to be viewed as a short-term solution for financial dilemmas. However, 85% of the HMOs contacted by *Modern HealthCare* stated that there is an immediate improvement in the quality of care provided patients (Manthey, 1988).

Commonalities

In reviewing the various models of case management, there appear to be several common threads:

- enhancement of care quality
- elimination of service duplication
- establishment of control over patient flow among all the services in an institution
- movement of patients out of costly inpatient beds to appropriate alternative care settings

CONCLUSION

Nurses are in the ideal position to facilitate the achievement of a balance between the issues of cost and quality. They have moved from being manual skill workers to being knowledge workers who have the competence to resolve the ethical dilemma of what to do and what not to do when there is more work than time available. They are able to use physician-specified patterns of care in conjunction with cost accounting and nursing knowledge and expertise to deliver cost-effective, quality patient care. They can facilitate the allocation of resources without compromising quality (Clifford & Plomann, 1985). Cost and quality can and *must* live together. Nurse managers and staff nurses have the opportunity and ability to ensure the balancing of cost and quality for patients and health care providers, by establishing and monitoring standards that measure productivity and quality outcomes. Through the development and implementation of a nursing care delivery system that incorporates these standards, consumer satisfaction can be achieved. Nursing is the catalyst that allows cost and quality to be compatible, and as a result allows health care providers to be successful.

REFERENCES

Beyers, M. (1986). Cost and quality: Balancing the issues through management. *Journal of Nursing Quality Assurance, 1*, 47–54.

Blaney, D.R., Hobson, C.J., & McHenry, J. (1988). Improving the cost effectiveness of nursing practice in an hospital setting. *Journal of Continuing Education in Nursing, 19*, 113–117.

Clemenhagen, C. (1987). Interplay between cost and quality. *Quality Review Bulletin, 87*, 138–139.

Clifford, L.A., & Plomann, M.P. (1985). Cost and quality: Two sides of the coin in cost containment. *HealthCare Financial Management, 39*, 30–32.

Collins, H.L. (1988). When the profit motive threatens patient care. *RN, 5*, 74–80.

Crane, M. (1986). How badly are cost controls hurting patients? *Medical Economics, 63*, 61–64.

Crisham, P. (1986). Ethics, economics, and quality. *Journal of Nursing Quality Assurance, 1*, 26–35.

Currie, E. (1987). Climate of negligence. *Nursing Times, 83*, 60.

Curtin, L.L. (1986). Editorial opinion: Who says "Lean" must be "Mean." *Nursing Management, 17*, 7–8.

Del Togno-Armanasco, V., Olivas, G., & Harter, S. (1989). Developing an integrated nursing case management model. *Nursing Management, 20*, 26–29.

Donabedian, A. (1984). Quality, cost, and cost containment. *Nursing Outlook, 32*, 142–145.

Donabedian, A. (1988). Quality and cost: Choices and responsibilities. *Inquiry, 25*, 90–99.

Ethridge, P. (1989). Unprofitable services turned profitable. *Health care strategic management, 7*, 5–6.

Everett, G.D. (1985). Quality assurance and cost containment in teaching hospitals: Implications for a period of economic restraint. *Quality Review Bulletin, 11*, 42–46.

Fisher, K. (1987). QA update: Case management. *Quality Review Bulletin, 13*, 287–290.

Fralic, M.F. (1988). Tracking cost while keeping quality alive (and well). *Journal of Nursing Administration, 18*, 7–8.

Fuchs, V.R. (1981). What is cost benefit analysis/cost effectiveness analysis, and why are they doing this to us? *New England Journal of Medicine, 303*, 937–938.

Gillis, D.M. (1987). Future directions: A business perspective. In *1987 Invitational Conference, National Commission on Nursing Implementation Project* (pp. 30–35). San Diego, CA.

Gordinier, R.H. (1985). Guest editorial: Purveyors of cost-containment, beware. *Postgraduate Medicine, 78*, 15–16.

Grif Alspach, J. (1986). Editorial: Reader survey report: Effects of cost-cutting measures on critical care nursing. *Critical Care Nurse, 6*, 1, 8–10.

Gross, K.F. (1986). A quality and cost control model for managing nursing utilization. *Journal of Nursing Quality Assurance, 1*, 36–46.

Hegyvary, S.T. (1988). *Research on strategies for maintaining quality in the delivery of patient care.* State-of-the-Science Invitational Conference: Nursing Resources and the Delivery of Patient Care: National Center for Nursing Research, February 18–19, 1988. Washington, DC: U.S. Department of Health and Human Services. (NIH Publication No. 89-3008, pp. 19–20).

Helt, E.H., & Jelinek, R.C. (1988). In the wake of cost cutting, nursing productivity and quality improve. *Nursing Management*, 36–39, 46–48.

Hoffman, F. (1988). *Nursing productivity assessment and costing out nursing services*. Philadelphia: JB Lippincott.

Jensen, J.C. (1988). Quality in health care: Marketers integrate the customer perspective. *Matrix, 1*, 4–6.

Kenkel, P.J. (1985). HMOs say gatekeeper system cuts costs, boosts quality. *Modern Healthcare, 15*, 6.

Kimball, M.C. (1990). Nation's health bill to rise 10.4% in 1990, U.S. says. *HealthWeek, 4*, 1, 52.

Krueger Wilson, C. (1986). Strategies for monitoring the cost and quality of care. *Journal of Nursing Quality Assurance, 1*, 55–65.

Larson, E.L., & Peters, D.A. (1986). Integrating cost analyses in quality assurance. *Journal of Nursing Quality Assurance, 1*, 1–7.

Lewis, E.M., Nitta, D.E., Biczi, T., & Robinson, M.A. (1986). Downsizing: Measuring its effects on quality of care. *Journal of Nursing Quality Assurance, 1*, 17–25.

Manthey, M. (1988). Cutbacks and shrinkages: A means to eliminate the "victim mentality." *Nursing Management, 17*, 17–18.

Mushlin, A.I. (1984). Measuring cost and quality of care under prospective reimbursement. *The Hospital Medical Staff, 13*, 17–21.

National Commission on Nursing Implementation Project. (1988). *Features of high quality, cost-effective nursing care delivery systems of the future*.

O'Donnell, W.E., Griffith, J.L., Donnell, J.M., Fuchs, B.C., Jencks, S.F., Doan, J.E., & Nestler, W.B. (1986). How badly is cost-containment hurting patient care? *Medical Economics, 63*, 48–64.

Omachonu V.K., & Nanda, R. (1989). Measuring productivity: Outcome vs. output. *Nursing Management, 20*, 35–40.

Panniers, T.L. (1987). Severity of illness, quality of care, and physician practice as determinants of hospital resource consumption. *Quality Review Bulletin, 13*, 158–165.

Rhea, J.T. (1986). Long-term improvement in cost and quality within hospitals. *Hospital & Health Services Administration*, 64–73.

Skydell, B., & Arndt, M. (1988). The price of nursing care. *Nursing Clinics of North America, 23*, 493–501.

Spitzer, R., & Priselac, T.M. *Nursing Productivity: The Hospital's Key to Survival and Profit*. Chicago: S-N Publications.

Syron, E.P., & Corey, H.J. (1989). Is monitoring money more important than monitoring quality? *Journal of Quality Assurance, 11*, 12–18.

VanderVeen, L.M. (1988). Cost containment and the link to quality. *Health Care Strategic Management, 6*, 13–21.

Yeater, D.C. (1984). Are you keeping up with health care cost containment management strategies? *Occupational Health Nursing, 32*, 193–198.

Zander, K. (1988). Managed care within acute care settings: Design and implementation via nursing case management. *Health Care Supervisor, 6*, 27–43.

4

Nursing Quality Assurance Programs: Unit-Based Nursing Quality Assurance Models

Patricia Schroeder, MSN, RN, Nursing Quality Consultant, Quality Care Concepts, Inc., Thiensville, Wisconsin

Unit-based nursing quality assurance (UBQA) has been considered a valuable and viable model for the conduct of quality assurance (QA) activities since 1982 (Schroeder, Maibusch, Anderson, & Formella, 1982). As the title suggests, UBQA is a decentralized approach to QA, with responsibility for the conduct of QA activities resting at the level of the nursing unit. An underlying tenet is that professional staff nurses are accountable for practice (Schroeder, 1988). Such accountability can only be accomplished through meaningful collaboration between staff nurses and nurse managers, since each brings unique perspectives, information, and skills to the program. Measures of the success of the program include improvement in patient care, involvement of professional staff nurses in decision making for practice, and achievement of the QA expectations of accrediting agencies (Schroeder, 1990).

The involvement of professional staff nurses in QA activities is well supported in the literature. Smeltzer, Hinshaw, and Feltman (1987) studied whether nurses who participate in QA activities possessed certain characteristics and whether they perceived the provision of their care differently from the way colleagues uninvolved in QA activities perceived it. Nurses involved in QA had higher levels of education than uninvolved nurses had and were more motivated to return to school. They differed significantly in their increased involvement in professional education. When asked to rate their perception of the level of care they commonly delivered, involved nurses rated their care at a higher level than uninvolved nurses rated theirs. Kraft, Neubauer, and LeSage (1987) describe the development and use of a QA monitoring tool for long-term care but suggest that its accurate use is based on involvement of professional nurses with a background in practice in the specialty of long-term care. They believe that professional decision making and the use of professional judgment are necessary for participation in QA activities.

Beyerman (1987) suggests that UBQA programs will not be successful unless the concept of decentralization is valued and demonstrated in a variety of ways

43

within the organization. If nurses believe that authority for practice rests with someone other than themselves, they will be hesitant to participate. Beyerman also states that the staff nurse's presence at the bedside allows for efficiency in data collection and facilitates problem resolution because of the nurse's resulting greater awareness of the issues.

Neubauer, Begley, Jankowski, and Keller (1988) describe the development and implementation of a comprehensive decentralized QA program in a large medical center. The authors state that the program has resulted in increased staff nurse ownership of unit-level QA issues, creating a sense of increased professional responsibility. "Responsible participation has resulted in nurses having increased control over clinical practice, a more meaningful work life, a renewed respect for peers, and a renewed commitment to the improvement of nursing care" (Neubauer et al., 1988, p. 7).

Thompson, Hylka, and Shaw (1988) describe the impact of staff nurse participation in a decentralized nursing QA program. Objectively, results of quality monitoring suggest that care has improved substantially, based on the QA program. Subjectively, staff nurse participants state that they have grown professionally from their involvement, and while the time to participate is difficult to find, they still choose to be involved because of the professional benefits. Staff nurses also reported that they received many positive comments from patients who appreciated and benefited from their interview-style data collection.

Many authors have also described benefits of staff nurse participation in decentralized nursing QA programs (Coyne & Killien, 1987; Crockett & Sutcliffe, 1986; Harris, Kreger, & Davis, 1989; Hendrickson, 1990; Kelly, 1984; O'Brien, 1988; Schroeder, 1984; Schroeder et al., 1982; Simpson & Sears, 1985). Participation, however, cannot be addressed as a single consistent activity, the same in all programs and achieving all good things. There is a distinct difference in the process and the outcomes of participation that equates with busywork (an activity for which professional nursing knowledge and skill are not required) and participation that is grounded in professional accountability and decision making. Underlying the accounts of positive benefits of staff nurse participation in decentralized QA programs are descriptions of the empowerment of professional nurses. Professional staff nurses in these agencies have been empowered to define expectations for practice and care, measure their achievement, and innovate to create improvements. It is inaccurate to speak of the same positive outcomes if the role of staff nurses in the QA program is merely that of data collectors not expected to plan, analyze, take action, and follow-up with clinical evaluation activities.

People are empowered by three key things: information, support, and resources (Moss Kanter, 1979). Information must include the mission, goals, and expectations of the organization. Organizational culture must be understood before one can expect to create change. The quality assurance/improvement process and program must be clearly defined so as to allow understanding. Clinical information and provision of available and useful data regarding practice and its environment are necessary before nurses can participate in the improvement of practice and care.

Support is also necessary for empowerment. Building quality into the role of the professional nurse requires readjustment of roles currently held. In order to successfully implement these processes, nurses must be supported by managers, by peers, and by the organization as a whole. There must be visible support and tolerance for flexibility, creativity, and failure. Education, guidance, and the help of resource people must be provided in an effort to ensure success.

Resources also play a role in empowerment. In health care settings, money, time, and expertise are valued. Meaningful involvement of professional nurses in a decentralized QA program requires all three. Nurses must be supported in carrying out QA activities on paid time. Quality-related activities and programs must be supported within department budgets. Industries outside of health care support such activities with specified budget allocations; this has not routinely happened in health care. It is necessary that QA be sufficiently valued to be financially supported. Ultimately, the cost of quality care is much less than the cost and potential liability risks of poor quality care.

Quality must be rewarded. This could take the form of rewarding the achievement of positive outcomes, the decrease in negative occurrences, the identification of a quality innovation that results in cost savings, or the negotiation for and the conduct of an innovative care activity that goes beyond one's commonly accepted role. Health care literature is only just beginning to identify programs designed to financially reward professionals for quality, beyond traditional performance appraisal and career ladders based on performance.

Approaches to quality improvement used in industries outside of health care support the importance of QA involvement of those carrying out the work of the organization. Such approaches and philosophies emphasize building quality into everyone's role and keeping decision making for quality improvement at the level closest to the actual service or production. The UBQA model parallels such a structure.

Models described as unit based have been implemented using a variety of structures and incorporating differing functions and roles. No single structure can be considered ultimately correct, given that many have been tailored to meet the needs and abilities of the organization and its professional staff.

Several variables affect structure. First, the functional definition of QA activities is not the same in all institutions. A definition is necessary to specify exactly what activities will be carried out at the unit level. These might include standards development and implementation, identification of major clinical functions, monitoring of care, analysis of monitoring data, implementation of actions to improve practice, risk management activities, ongoing education, input into peer evaluation, nurse privileging and credentialing, and so on. Some UBQA programs have a narrow and specific focus, while others are broad and incorporate many clinical issues and activities.

A second differentiating variable is the structure used at the unit level to carry out QA activities. Many approaches have been used to plan and identify responsibilities. Schroeder (1988) describes a model in which each unit has a QA committee comprised of staff nurses, the head nurse, and a clinical nurse specialist facilitator. Neubauer et al. (1988) discuss a decentralized QA program in a large medical center that functioned through the work of one staff nurse QA facilitator on each unit and a QA coordinator for each clinical service. Other staff nurses were integrated into activities at the unit level. Some agencies have incorporated responsibility for QA into the role of the head nurse, who then delegates activities to other nurses as he or she is able. Still other agencies have created multidisciplinary QA committees to carry out QA at the unit level. Structures continue to evolve into many different forms.

The structure of UBQA at the unit level is ultimately affected by the third variable: How it will be coordinated across the clinical service or department. Variations in models occur based on whether some QA activities are centralized (i.e., department-wide versus unit-specific standards and monitoring activities, responsibility for corrective actions, etc.), where decisions about practice and innovation can be made (degree of bureaucracy), the extent to which units are encouraged to collaborate with other departments (departmental boundaries), and the responsible body (person or committee) for coordinating QA activities across the department. Again, there is no single correct approach that can be identified, as many have been successful.

In addition to these variables specific to the structure of the QA program, however, several other elements are necessary for the successful implementation of any QA model or approach. These elements are essential, irrespective of the particular ideology espoused.

An organizational commitment to quality must be present and must be emphasized by the leaders of the organization. Staff members must believe that the organization is committed to its mission and to the delivery of a quality product or service. The quality program cannot be seen as a fad or as a program with which the organization will lose interest. Everyone within the organization must value quality in visible and action-oriented ways. Quality must be given constant attention and ultimate importance.

A viable quality program must be created. Some suggest that any program can be effective as long as it is practical, sincere, and enduring. To be viable, the quality program must fit with the way the organization does business. It must match the organizational culture and the staff. It must be based on the resources available and allocated. Too many QA programs look glorious on paper but create frustration in staffs who know that they cannot possibly be implemented in their organization's current state.

Finally, staff involved in the QA program must be empowered to carry out their roles. Decision making for practice, creating innovations, and precipitating organizational change are serious and significant issues within the health care setting. People cannot be told simply to "do it" without being educated, prepared, and supported in the process. Once learned, these skills can be applied to other aspects of the professional role. The potential of an empowered staff is unfathomable.

Overall, approaches to successfully implement a UBQA program vary dramatically in their structure, functions, and outcomes. Given the wide variation, one is left to wonder whether UBQA can, in fact, be considered a specific model, or whether instead this label has been coined to typify philosophic premises about health care quality–related programs.

UBQA has become synonymous with staff nurse accountability for QA. Care must be taken not to assume that the shifting of responsibility for QA from a central source to the unit level, or from an administrator to a staff member, will guarantee success. It is not enough to take the quality efforts to the unit if they never reach the bedside. The premise and true spirit of the UBQA approach fits with other QA models and quality improvement philosophies. UBQA can be a strategy to build quality into the service and product of health care, instead of inspecting for quality only after the fact. To the extent that this spirit is integrated into other models, the distinctiveness of the UBQA model becomes blurred. Then, its benefits remain, and our capacity to deliver quality health care moves forward.

REFERENCES

Beyerman, K. (1987). Developing a unit-based nursing quality assurance program: From concept to practice. *Journal of Nursing Quality Assurance, 2,* 1–11.

Coyne, C., & Killien, M. (1987). A system for unit-based monitors of quality of nursing care. *Journal of Nursing Administration, 17,* 26–32.

Crockett, D., & Sutcliffe, S. (1986). Staff participation in nursing quality assurance. *Nursing Management, 17,* 41–42.

Harris, S.H., Kreger, S.M., & Davis, M.Z. (1989). A problem-focused quality assurance program. *Nursing Management, 20,* 54–60.

Hendrickson, S.W. (1990). Implementing a unit-based quality assurance program. *Journal of Nursing Quality Assurance, 4,* 7–17.

Kelly, P. (1984). Differentiating roles in quality assurance. *Dimensions of Critical Care Nursing, 3,* 104–109.

Kraft, M.R., Neubauer, J.A., & LeSage, J. (1987). Quality monitoring in long term care. *Journal of Nursing Quality Assurance, 2,* 39–48.

Moss Kanter, R.M. (1979). Power failure in management circuits. *Harvard Business Review, 57,* 65–75.

Neubauer, J.A., Begley, B., Jankowski, B.Z., & Keller, K. (1988). Development and implementation of unit-based monitors. *Journals of Nursing Quality Assurance, 2,* 1–8.

O'Brien, B. (1988). QA: A commitment to excellence. *Nursing Management, 19,* 33–34, 38–40.

Schroeder, P. (1984). The quality assurance process. In P. Schroeder & R. Maibusch (Eds.), *Nursing quality assurance: A unit-based approach* (pp. 79–93). Gaithersburg, MD: Aspen Publishers.

Schroeder, P. (1988). UBQA: The system revisited. In S.E. Pinkerton & P. Schroeder (Eds.), *Commitment to excellence: Developing a professional nursing staff* (pp. 33–41). Gaithersburg, MD: Aspen Publishers.

Schroeder, P. (1990). From the editor. *Journal of Nursing Quality Assurance, 4,* vii–viii.

Schroeder, P., Maibusch, R., Anderson, C., & Formella, N. (1982). A unit-based approach to nursing quality assurance. *Quality Review Bulletin, 8,* 10–12.

Simpson, K., & Sears, R. (1985). Authority and responsibility delegation predicts quality of care. *Journal of Advanced Nursing, 10,* 345–348.

Smeltzer, C., Hinshaw, A.S., & Feltman, B. (1987). The benefits of staff nurse involvement in monitoring the quality of patient care. *Journal of Nursing Quality Assurance, 1,* 1–7.

Thompson, M.W., Hylka, S.C., & Shaw, C.F. (1988). Systematic monitoring of generic standards of patient care. *Journal of Nursing Quality Assurance, 2,* 9–15.

5

Integration of Quality Assurance in a Decentralized Organization

Jo Marie Walrath, MS, RN, Director of Nursing, Surgery, The Johns Hopkins Hospital, Baltimore, Maryland

Karen B. Haller, PhD, RN, Director of Nursing, Research and Education, The Johns Hopkins Hospital, Baltimore, Maryland

Linda M. Arenth, MS, RN, Vice President for Nursing and Patient Services, The Johns Hopkins Hospital, Baltimore, Maryland

Carol M. Beekman, MSN, RN, Nursing Staff Assistant, Surgery, The Johns Hopkins Hospital, Baltimore, Maryland

The culture in a decentralized hospital places a high value on local autonomy and authority, with decision making being concentrated closest to the point of clinical service. The philosophy behind a quality assurance (QA) program that puts the emphasis at the unit level is highly compatible with the values of a decentralized institution.

Problem resolution occurs at two levels within a decentralized QA program: the hospital level and the unit level. The challenge for QA programs in decentralized hospitals is to develop the type of cooperative relationships that permit integration of efforts across both levels and among health care providers. A successful QA program in such an environment must provide for communication flow in all directions (Saum, 1988, p. 19).

This chapter discusses the tenets of decentralized management, describes the decentralized organization in place at The Johns Hopkins Hospital, and explores the integration of QA activities within a decentralized institution.

THE TENETS OF DECENTRALIZED MANAGEMENT

Decentralized management models were widespread in industry before their adoption by some hospitals, primarily during the 1970s (Drucker, 1973). Historically, hospitals have been managed by a series of vertical structures, with little decision making delegated to the level where the work was being done. Under this traditional model, for example, there is a strong central nursing department responsible for nursing practice throughout the hospital. Personnel and budgetary decisions are made centrally.

Decentralization shifts operating responsibility and fiscal accountability in hospitals to clinical departments. Central management reserves control only over what technologies or markets to develop, what services to provide or abandon, the management and allocation of capital, and the selection of key managers and professionals (Drucker, 1974).

Drucker (1973) has described two forms of decentralization: federal decentralization and simulated decentralization. In federal models, the company or hospital is organized into a number of autonomous businesses. Each unit has responsibility for its own performance and contribution to the company. Simulated decentralization is used as a management system when a business cannot be set up as an autonomous unit, because its size and complexity contributes to managerial ineffectiveness. In this model, structural units are set up as businesses with all possible autonomy and their own management, but with "simulation" of profit-and-loss responsibility. With both models, the major purposes of decentralization are to improve the responsiveness of the institution to changes in its environment and to strengthen overall management of the organization.

DECENTRALIZATION: THE MODEL AT THE JOHNS HOPKINS HOSPITAL

The Johns Hopkins Hospital implemented a federal decentralization model in 1973 (Heyssel, Gaintner, Kues, Jones, & Lipstein, 1984). The hospital was reorganized into functional management units. These functional units are organized along major clinical service lines such as pediatrics, medicine, and surgery, in effect making the hospital a holding company for a group of specialty hospitals. While the hospital maintains a framework of common policy and mutually set goals, each functional unit has its own budget and plan of operations. Central management personnel have staff roles without line responsibilities for operations. Conversely, maximum autonomy and responsibility for financial, operational, and programmatic issues are delegated to the functional units.

Nursing in the Decentralized Model

The nursing organization has both central and departmental functions and structures. The vice president for nursing and patient services is accountable for professional nursing practice and standards. Responsibility for QA, education, research, professional nursing recruitment, and the overall compensation program is vested in the vice president's office. These responsibilities are managed through an active QA program, effective management information systems, and function-specific committees with representatives from the clinical departments. Directors of nursing in the clinical units have responsibility for managing all departmental nursing programs and all nursing personnel, as well as for budgeting resources. As a result, fiscal and operational responsibilities are concentrated in the functional units, while accountability for nursing practice and standards is maintained centrally. This structure ensures a unified direction for nursing across the institution yet promotes diversity and innovation within the units.

Nursing QA

Because responsibility for nursing QA rests with the vice president for nursing and patient services, a hospital-wide program that includes all nursing divisions within functional units was set up to establish and maintain both the structure and the process for ensuring excellent nursing care. There is a parallel structure and process for nursing QA in each of the functional units, where accountability for identification and resolution of problems ultimately rests. The functions of the hospital-wide nursing QA program and a functional unit program will be presented below. The department of surgery will be used to exemplify the integration of the central nursing program with a departmental program.

NURSING QA: THE HOSPITAL-WIDE PROGRAM

The QA program for the entire department of nursing is charged with setting generic standards and developing and implementing the means to monitor and evaluate universal components of practice. Resolution of identified problems rests with the functional unit. In addition, the central program must integrate the efforts of nursing with those of other disciplines.

Structure

The hospital-wide department of nursing's QA program is designed to integrate the efforts of all eight functional units (departments). The director of nursing from each sits on the QA steering committee, along with the vice president for nursing and patient services. By having the directors make up the steering committee, duplication of effort is avoided, and problem tracking and resolution are also enhanced. The director of QA, a central staff person, chairs the steering committee and is accountable for overall program administration; however, department directors have the responsibility for implementing practice changes on their units. The QA program is implemented using a central committee structure that incorporates five committees, respectively charged with responsibility for (1) standards of practice, (2) standards of care, (3) monitoring and evaluation, (4) staff education, and (5) research. All of these functions are essential to ensure that the patient receives quality nursing care. The structural components of this model are shown in Figure 5-1.

All departments have one representative on each of the five committees. This allows all clinical areas' concerns to be raised in a central forum and facilitates problem solving by making the expertise of the whole institution available to single units. Representatives are appointed to committees by their respective directors of nursing. These appointments consider the expertise of the individuals. For example, members of the staff with doctoral education tend to be appointed to the research committee, clinical instructors to the staff education committee, and expert practitioners in a variety of roles to the standards of care committee.

Process

The QA steering committee has four main purposes:

1. provide a structure and process that ensures documentation and appropriate communication of nursing QA activities
2. provide a means for problem resolution (identification, assessment, intervention, and monitoring)
3. ensure the clinical competence and promote the professional development of nursing staff through education and evaluation
4. ensure excellent care, delivered in a cost-efficient manner, for all patients

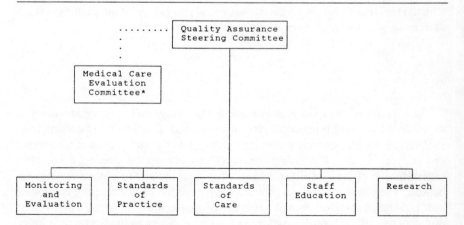

Figure 5-1 Department of Nursing QA Committees. *Source:* Reprinted with permission from The Johns Hopkins Hospital, *Nursing Practice and Organization Manual*, 1989.

*Integration point of nursing and all other department quality assurance programs.

Specific goals for the QA steering committee are mutually set by the directors of nursing during the department of nursing's annual strategic planning process. Thus the QA program is an integral part of the larger plan for professional nursing at Hopkins.

Communication

The QA steering committee meets monthly to fulfill its functions and achieve its goals. At this meeting, each of the five program committees gives a formal report. This mechanism allows directors to synthesize details on the diverse components of the program and assimilate this information into their unit-based programs. Similarly, the meeting provides directors with an opportunity to enrich the central program by identifying mutual problems, sharing unit data, and suggesting avenues for resolving problems.

All of the central committees are chaired by a director who sits on the steering committee. Thus the central committees have an opportunity to "talk" to one another during the steering meetings. This dialogue between chairpersons ensures maximum coordination and integration of efforts. For example, the monitoring and evaluation committee identified insufficient documentation of the nursing process in the medical record as a problem shared by more than half of the departments. They recommended that head nurse education be offered on both documentation and a peer-auditing process by which head nurses could assist their staff to be accountable for the nursing process. The staff education committee subsequently organized this educational program, using the expertise of two units that had successfully implemented peer-auditing and self-auditing of nursing process documentation.

Nurses who sit on the five committees that make up the central QA structure gain heightened awareness of the hospital-wide nursing concerns. They have a responsibility to communicate this understanding to their units, just as they have a responsibility to interpret the uniqueness of their departments' needs to the larger nursing community at Hopkins. Thus the two-way communication between nursing units and the entire department of nursing is dependent on both directors and central committee members.

Problem Resolution

Problems may be identified by any individual or group within the institution. Knowledge of the problem may enter the QA program at the central or the department level. Departmental issues are routed to the steering committee in the monthly meetings. It is at this point that the steering committee chair either assigns it to the appropriate nursing subcommittee for analysis and resolution or links into a more appropriate forum within the hospital committee structure.

The hospital-wide nursing QA program diligently monitors selected high-risk, high-volume, or problem-prone areas of care. The goal is to identify potential problems and design preventive strategies. Responsibility for identifying areas of common concern and implementing the audit is given to the monitoring and evaluation committee. For example, when a new policy on universal precautions was adopted by the hospital, educational programs were instituted. The department of nursing needed to know if the inservice education was sufficient to prevent needle sticks; therefore, the monitoring and evaluation committee conducted an audit of compliance with the policy and monitored the number of sticks reported to the personnel health advisor. In this audit, as all other audits of generic quality indicators, the data are gathered by the units and analyzed per unit. This permits each functional area to determine whether it has a problem and to tailor interventions to its specific situation.

Development of Nursing Staff

Educational programs required as a result of audit findings are coordinated and offered centrally by the staff education committee. These have included such diverse topics as respiratory care, universal precautions, standards of care, and standards of practice.

Excellent Care

The assurance of uniform care throughout the hospital rests on the implementation of generic standards of practice and standards of care. These standards set the minimum expectation of care. A committee develops, implements, and maintains each of these sets of standards. At this time, Hopkins is making the transition from monitoring the process of care to monitoring the outcome of care. This should allow the identification of nursing interventions that do not appear to be effective, even when implemented well. It is expected that outcome evaluation will raise questions about traditional nursing interventions and move the research committee toward outcome research.

NURSING QA: DEPARTMENTAL PROGRAMS

A structure and process exists in each department for organizing, implementing, and monitoring the quality of nursing care. The design of the program varies from area to area, consistent with Hopkins' decentralized model; therefore, the program in one clinical division, the department of surgery, will be presented to exemplify the integration of nursing QA activities across the institution.

The nursing division within the department of surgery consists of 23 operating suites, a recovery room, 3 intensive care units, 9 inpatient units, outpatient clinics, and a "same-day surgery" center. The specialization within the department challenges the staff's ability to integrate QA into a meaningful program.

Structure

The overall purpose of the QA program within the department is to ensure optimal patient care for surgical patients. The program is organized, implemented, and monitored by a steering committee that has four working subcommittees. This departmental committee structure design differs from the central program, although the committees' functions, goals, and expected outcomes parallel those of the hospital-wide nursing QA program (see Table 5-1).

It is at the nursing unit level within the department that the structure of the surgical nursing QA program differs from the central hospital. Three unit-based committees exit on each nursing unit: (1) clinical practice, (2) nursing education, and (3) monitoring and evaluation. These committees are chaired by senior clinical nurses who report committee recommendations to the nurse manager on the units. The functions of each of these committees are detailed in Table 5-2.

Operating a unit-based QA program supports the hospital's management philosophy that accountability needs to be placed in the hands of those who are at the operational level. It is the expert practicing nurse who is given the responsibility for defining excellent nursing care on the unit, developing appropriate mechanisms to ensure the delivery of high-quality care, and monitoring the outcomes of nursing practice. Accountability for redressing nursing care problems is also placed in the hands of the nurse.

Process

The Division of Surgical Nursing's steering committee is where all nursing QA activities are integrated. The primary functions of this committee are to

1. review monthly all incidents and their trends, QA committee reports, audit results, and nursing practice issues and events
2. set priorities for any QA topics to be monitored that have general applicability across the department
3. evaluate the overall effectiveness of the QA program

Table 5-1 Department of Surgery QA Committees

Committee	Functions
Steering committee	• Establishes direction and priority of departmental quality assurance activities. • Integrates hospital-wide nursing quality assurance program with departmental efforts. • Disseminates approved policies, procedures, and protocols.
Standards of care and documentation	• Serves as a resource for development of unit based standards of care and protocols. • Reviews new or revised documentation forms for submission to hospital documentation committee. • Recommends refinements or revisions to department clinical documentation system. • Maintains state of the art patient discharge instruction information.
Monitoring and evaluation	• Provides forum for communication and coordination of central departmental and unit based monitoring activities. • Serves as a resource for unit based committee members in the area of tool development and data evaluation.
Policy and procedure	• Reviews submitted policies and procedures for compliance with standards set by hospital and regulatory agencies. • Acts in an advisory capacity to unit based committees in the area of policy procedure development.
Research and staff education	• Recommends educational programs or research efforts needed to address identified problems from hospital or departmental quality assurance efforts.

Source: Courtesy of The Johns Hopkins Hospital, Department of Surgical Nursing, Baltimore, MD.

4. modify the QA program as needed
5. disseminate all new standards, policies, procedures, or clinical protocols
6. establish appropriate task forces to address issues that fall outside of the current committee structure
7. serve as a resource to the standing committees

A wide variety of clinical and administrative issues emerge from departmental and unit-based QA activities. To respond expeditiously to problems and preserve the integrity of the program requires effective communication. Unit committees report through their nurse managers to the department's steering committee. In turn, the director of nursing can convey specific unit concerns to the central committee. Additional communication between the departmental and hospital pro-

Table 5-2 Committee Structure on Nursing Units

Committee	Purpose
Clinical practice	• Identify and make recommendations regarding clinical practice issues, environmental, or organizational barriers that adversely affect the delivery of patient care. • Develop unit based standards, protocols, policies or procedures that are specific to the patient population managed on the unit.
Nursing education	• Conduct an assessment which identifies staff or patient educational needs. • Implement and evaluate all unit specific educational programs for both staff and patients. • Monitor compliance to required department educational updates e.g., risk management, CPR.
Monitoring and evaluation	• Identify high volume, high risk, problem-prone practice issues that are specific to the patient population or unit. • Conduct studies of identified problems. • Analyze results of monitoring activities and recommend corrective action. • Evaluate effectiveness of corrective action and submit final report.

Note: CPR = cardiopulmonary resuscitation.

Source: Courtesy of The Johns Hopkins Hospital, Department of Surgical Nursing, Baltimore, MD.

grams is facilitated by having the chairpersons of the subcommittees serve as members of the central hospital committees. For example, the chair of the department's staff education committee is a member of the hospital-wide staff education committee.

INTEGRATION OF CENTRALIZED AND DECENTRALIZED FUNCTIONS

A concerted effort is made to balance hospital-wide, departmental, and unit needs when determining QA goals and objectives. This effort is made within nursing, as well as among nursing and other disciplines.

Integration of Nursing QA Activities

The central QA program selects for review one or two critical indicators annually. These indicators have applicability across all the functional units. Topics such as informed discharge, documentation of the nursing process, and universal precautions have been selected in the past. The hospital program is moving toward selection of outcome standards as generic indicators in the future. In the department of surgery, topics such as postoperative pain management, wound care, and aseptic technique have been selected for focused reviews because they are specific to the practice of surgical nursing.

Integration of Nursing QA with Other Disciplines

Nursing's QA programs are coordinated with the initiatives of other health professionals at both the departmental level and the hospital level. Each department has an interdisciplinary QA committee, of which nursing is a key member. Information may flow down to these committees from central nursing or come up from the other disciplines to nursing's attention. Each of these departmental interdisciplinary committees has a "physician advisor" who is responsible for medical QA. In a similar position to the nursing member, the physician advisor may take information up the ranks to the central medical evaluation committee, which in turn reports to the medical board; conversely, information flows from the medical board through the medical evaluation committee to the physician advisors. These relationships and the resultant flow of information are shown in Figure 5-2.

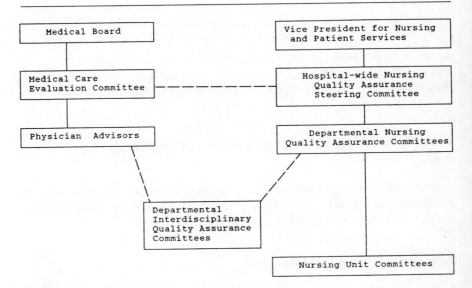

Figure 5-2 Coordination of QA Activities

Figure 5-2 also demonstrates the coordination between the central coordinating bodies for both nursing and medicine. The nursing QA steering committee has a joint member of the medical care evaluation committee and makes a formal report at the meeting of the medical committee. Since respiratory therapy, pharmacy, infection control, and a number of other disciplines are organized as subcommittees of the medical care evaluation committee, nursing's participation provides an opportunity to integrate its efforts with those being made by other disciplines. As a result, The Johns Hopkins Hospital can assure the patient that excellent care is being rendered.

MANAGING ONGOING CHALLENGES IN QA

In a decentralized system, responsibility and accountability for QA are also decentralized. Authority for ensuring excellent care is assigned at the operating level where practitioners can identify problems early and make the requisite changes. Those staff most closely associated with the problem are involved in monitoring and resolving the issue.

The major advantage to a decentralized program is that "quality" can be defined differently, but appropriately, in each operating unit. Similarly, the solutions to problems can be tailored to fit the needs of particular working environments or patient populations. These advantages are achieved by creating a complex system of organizational structures and processes, which necessitates an equally complex pattern of communications. Ensuring effective communication in all directions requires the commitment of all health care providers in the institution.

The challenge of communicating effectively is formidable, but the rewards are gratifying: A broad base of diverse views and opinions is considered in identifying problems, designing effective monitoring systems, and crafting solutions. Thus the model demonstrates the participatory management style that is essential in fully decentralized organizations. Because decentralization also encourages and fosters innovation, some departments may generate and test solutions to a problem before other units have yet identified the issue. A broader range of quality issues is tackled by allowing such diversity. The departmental and hospital-wide committees, both within nursing and between nursing and medicine, facilitate the sharing of ideas and prevent "reinvention of the wheel." By winnowing out redundant efforts across departments, more staff can turn their attention to specialized aspects of practice that can only be effectively addressed in their areas or with their patient populations. Therefore, the QA program in a decentralized system benefits from monitoring both generic issues and unit-specific activities.

REFERENCES

Drucker, P.W. (1973). *Management tasks, responsibilities, and practices.* New York: Harper & Row.

Drucker, P.W. (1974). *Management tasks, responsibilities, and practices* (2nd ed.). New York: Harper & Row.

Heyssel, R.M., Gaintner, J.R., Kues, I.W., Jones, A.A., & Lipstein, S.H. (1984). Decentralized management in a teaching hospital. *New England Journal of Medicine, 310*, 1477–1480.

Saum, M.F. (1988). Evaluation: A vital component of the quality assurance program. *Journal of Nursing Quality Assurance, 2*, 17–24.

6

The Marker Umbrella Model for Quality Assurance

Carolyn G. Smith Marker, RN, MSN, President, Marker Systems, Severna Park, Maryland

DEFINITION AND PHILOSOPHY

The Marker Umbrella Model for quality assurance (QA) is a practice model that defines the nine interdependent components of professional QA and focuses on a dual approach of active problem identification/resolution and compliance monitoring to structure, process, and outcome standards (Marker, 1989, p. 41).

The development and implementation of the model is based on seven philosophical values. First, QA is both a managerial and a staff responsibility. QA is done by managers because it is a vehicle for defining practice, an approach for data collection on which to base clinical and management decisions and corrective actions, and a powerful mechanism for holding self and staff accountable to safe, effective, and appropriate systems function, staff performance, and patient care. QA is participatively carried out by staff because it is an extension of the last step of the nursing process, evaluation of effectiveness. Staff evaluate the care of individual patients during a shift. For example, a registered nurse questions a patient about pain relief after administering pain medication. In unit-based QA activities the staff registered nurse evaluates pain management and relief on a number of patients on the unit being cared for by a variety of colleagues, thus practicing QA via peer review.

Second, QA can only be effective when it is carried out universally through a practice model defining common activities, methods, and tools.

Third, QA is composed of universal events, applicable to all professional disciplines. For QA to be truly professional, it must be comprehensive, complete, and produce comparable results. When QA is driven by a practice model and universal events, measurable change can be assessed equally across units, clinical divisions, and departments. There is no such thing as nursing QA or physician QA or pharmacy QA! The activities are the same; only the topics and approaches differ because obviously the clinical focus of each department is different.

Fourth, good QA evolves over time. All professionals who carry out evaluation activities must develop "C squared": competence and confidence. One has to learn what QA is and the creative techniques for practicing it. Because a variety of activities are necessary, time is essential to implement one activity at a time, build the program in successive increments, maintain it over time, evaluate it for effectiveness, and periodically adjust it based on results and changing external requirements.

Fifth, QA must be defined and practiced with a dual approach of problem resolution and standards compliance. Redundant activities reviewing limited or procedural aspects of practice lead to superficial findings and little sustained or meaningful change. Sixth, the evaluation of the effectiveness of QA is measured not in terms of volume of statistics accumulated, quantity of papers shuffled, amount of time invested, or degree of emotional commitment expended. Simply, QA is effective only when problems are proven resolved over time, measured standards are in consistent compliance, thresholds for evaluation (TFE) are controlled, and measurable improvement in systems function, staff performance, and patient care is documented.

Seventh, and finally, QA is inherent to professional practice. It is driven not by external agencies or bureaucratic demands but by aspirations of excellence internal to the health care facility and professional practitioner. Likewise, decisions about approaches, methods, tools, compliance factors, major clinical activities to be monitored, corrective action plans, criteria development, and data collection and reporting mechanisms are the prerogative of the practitioners and are determined by need, proven effectiveness, and ability to produce comparable results.

CHARACTERISTICS OF THE UMBRELLA MODEL

The Marker Umbrella Model for QA is a comprehensive, multifaceted, and sophisticated quality management system. It is reality oriented and encompasses both unit-based and department-wide strategies within nursing. The model is universally applicable to all departments because the nine activities are generic and integrated into a total package of defining, monitoring, evaluating, reporting, and professional accountability. The activities inherent to the QA mechanism provide a framework to promote managerial function as well as maximum staff involvement and clinical competency. Perhaps the model's most significant characteristic is synergism. Synergism means that the whole is greater than the sum of its parts. Many traditional QA programs involve limited activities that are isolated and fragmented. Frequently no two events are connected, and therefore the energy yielded from the activities is limited to that put into the activity! In systems theory, consider what happens to a system when output is only equal to input—it self-destructs because there is insufficient energy to sustain it! Or the energy to sustain the system is so great that it can only be drawn from the product, which then diminishes the output for limited input to begin the cycle again, and so forth.

MAJOR LIMITATION OF QA TODAY

This analogy seems to apply to the profession of nursing today: There is little synergism—a lot of energy input, but minimal productivity and satisfaction output. Certainly it appears to apply to QA. If all nursing departments are doing as much effective QA as they say they are; if the tons of QA literature written, conferences attended, and paper generated are being truly productive; if patient care improvement and nurse satisfaction are evident; then why the current nursing depression? Why the constant superficial changes in QA terminology by the surveying external agencies? And why the extremely high rate of "contingencies or recommendations" given by surveying agencies in the area of QA? It is high time that the profession of nursing take stock and collectively stop wasting time, money, and manpower. It is almost past time that nursing staff and leadership assume the serious responsibility of defining professional nursing via its structure, process, and outcome; delineating the component aspects of nursing systematically, as opposed to forcing all content into limited policy/procedure; differentiating nursing from medical and non-nursing clerical and technical duties; standardizing practice and care to deliver a consistent and continuous product to the consumer who needs it and pays for it; and, finally, validating professional nursing in terms of its worth, contribution, and effectiveness. All the above responsibilities can be achieved via practice models for standards and QA. Without practice models adopted universally by the professional, each nurse, department, and facility is left to do "its own thing." The subsequent inconsistency in both approach and results makes it virtually impossible to compare effectiveness from one nursing department to another. This in turn devalues the total QA effort through redundancy, wasted resources, and task-oriented behaviors.

DESCRIPTION OF NINE INDEPENDENT ACTIVITIES

The Marker Umbrella Model for QA diagrams nine activities of QA (see Figure 6-1). Each activity stands alone yet is interdependent with all the others. This total integration of QA events produces maximum program productivity, effectiveness, and synergy (Marker, 1988a).

Standards development is the base of all professional practice. Using the sister to the Umbrella Model, the Marker Model for Standards Development, each department and unit develops the structure standards for systems operation in the

Marker Umbrella Model for Quality Assurance

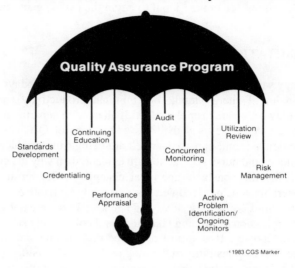

Figure 6-1 Marker Umbrella Model for QA. *Source:* © Carolyn G. Smith Marker, RN, MSN, 1983.

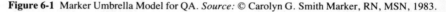

Process defines required practice behaviors as well as essential aspects of patient care, thus addressing both the nurse and the patient. There are six formats for process standards. Job descriptions define generic behaviors for a given level of worker. Performance standards expand these behaviors to the unit level to define a required level of competency. Procedures outline the technical aspects of nursing and are limited to psychomotor skills. Protocols define ongoing care/management of broad patient care problems in the areas of noninvasive and invasive equipment; therapeutic, diagnostic, and prophylactic management; temporary physiological/psychological states; and select nursing diagnoses. Guidelines define the use of documentation forms and tools. Standards of care are predefined care plans written for a patient population group having common problems and needs and may be in the style of standard care plans or statements, depending on the acuity of the patient and length of stay. Nursing diagnoses, patient outcomes, and precise interventions make up the standard of care. Interventions often encompass existing protocols to prevent redundancy. Outcome standards are written as goals and may be patient outcome–oriented, nursing goal–oriented, or both. Outcome standards are integrated into patient teaching protocols and standards of care; define physiological, psychological, and cognitive end states; and facilitate care planning, outcome audit, response-oriented nursing documentation, and discharge planning (see Figure 6-2) (Marker, 1988b, pp. 17–30).

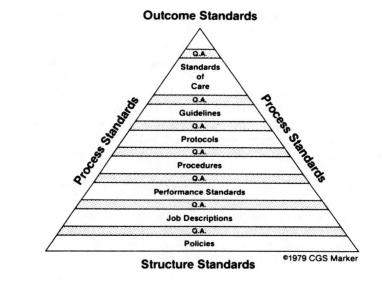

Figure 6-2 Marker model for standards development. *Source:* © Carolyn G. Smith Marker, RN, MSN, 1979.

The standards base provides content for criteria development and data retrieval for the major activities of audit and concurrent monitoring. Auditing is the formal process of data collection from a representative sample to judge compliance to a standard. It is done in three categories: (1) compliance reviews (six per year in the areas of structure, process, and outcome), (2) noncompliance reviews (done as often as required to pursue further investigation when TFEs are exceeded), and (3) miscellaneous reviews in the form of documentation studies; satisfaction surveys for patient, nursing staff, and physician feedback; occasional generic nursing review questionnaires; and mock Joint Commission on Accreditation of Healthcare Organizations (Joint Commission) surveys every 18 months.

In between the audit activities, concurrent monitoring takes place on the nursing unit a minimum of once per week. Concurrent monitoring involves staff members selecting major clinical activities and spot checking compliance via direct observation of care and performance. Since only one to four cases are observed at a time, this form of peer review is easily accepted by the staff, as it can be integrated into the unit routine without significant disruption to patient care, excessive time commitment, or overtime dollars. Both the audit (representative sample) and the concurrent monitor (spot checking) are based on predeveloped criteria using special criteria development sheets and a data retrieval form for consistency (Marker, 1988a, pp. 48–53).

Standards also form the base of the next three Umbrella events: continuing education, credentialing, and performance appraisal. Continuing education should occur in relation to three need areas: maintaining competency in relation to existing standards, creating competency in relation to newly developed standards, and responding to QA findings of noncompliance due to lack of knowledge and skill. Results of all continuing education should be linked to QA findings through increased compliance and/or effective problem resolution. Documentation of CE should be housed in the QA manual and be contained in three forms: continuing education events list, mandatory events list, and individual staff continuing education record. All events should be justified by reasons for the event as well as the impact of the event on performance and care.

Credentialing involves both licensure validation for legal competency and applied knowledge base and skill validation for professional competency in relation to existing generic and unit-specific standards. Documentation of credentialing is housed in the QA manual in three forms: annual licensure update, annual internal certification record, and clinical privileges approval list (Marker, 1987, pp. 58–59).

Performance appraisal represents another section of the QA manual; it contains an explanation of the appraisal system, including its approach, frequency, and relationship to standards and QA. The Umbrella Model advocates annual staff evaluation based on the generic job description. This annual evaluation is derived from ongoing performance monitoring via direct observation of staff function and anecdotal recording of compliance to predefined unit-based performance standards. Feedback is given on a quarterly basis to each staff member, which is then summarized at the end of the year. Information for ongoing performance monitoring is obtained from direct supervision of staff and from QA monitors. This is possible because the data retrieval form cross-references QA results with the caregiver. Thus QA directly affects performance ratings and pay for performance.

Utilization review (UR) comprises the seventh activity of QA. UR is an essential component that should be diagrammed under the QA umbrella instead of in the traditional side, competitive position. This is often demonstrated in QA literature as ''QA/UR/RM'' (RM = risk management). Utilization is a strategy of QA, not an unrelated or alternate event. UR is used to track and trend appropriate and effective use of human, fiscal, and physical resources, as well as to record the occurrence of negative events. A special section of the QA manual houses the UR tools. This includes the unit log for recording patient entry, origin of admission, primary/secondary diagnoses, length of stay, discharge data, disposition, and complications via generic screens. The generic screens encompass the Joint Commission housewide universal indicators, along with special indicators for the particular clinical area, such as the intensive care unit or psychiatry. This information is tracked on a daily basis and trended monthly on the utilization of the unit record. Fiscal data including average daily census, hours per patient day, average length of stay, and average acuity levels provide the manager with essential data for ongoing manipulation and control of fiscal resources. Volume indicators of adverse events such as falls, medication errors, wound infections, invasive device infections, skin breakdown, mortality rates, unsuccessful resuscitations, serious drug reactions, and so forth, can be immediately compared with thresholds for necessary further investigation.

RM is the eighth QA activity. RM events are directed at minimizing and controlling loss. The RM section of the QA manual contains five tools: safety reviews, both generic and unit-specific to the area, done on an every-other-quarter basis; infection control reviews, performed on alternate quarters and based on universal precautions and unit-specific requirements; emergency equipment/drug checks, done as required by the Joint Commission; preventive maintenance records, filled out monthly, including generic and unit-specific parameters; and incident tracking reports, completed monthly to track events posing a risk of litigation (Marker, 1987, pp. 61–62).

The final activity under the QA umbrella is active problem identification (API). The API component of QA is the most flexible and creative and involves the development and implementation of data collection tools for problem identification and resolution (PI/PR). These tools may be used on a shift, daily, weekly, monthly, or quarterly basis for data tracking and trending. They are completed by a variety of personnel, including the unit manager, staff nurses, unit secretary, charge/shift coordinator, physicians, and department heads. Two related tools are the problem identification sheet and the problem log. The former is used by any caregiver to record a known or potential problem that has or may interfere with safe, effective, and appropriate care or performance. Generally problems fall into seven categories: equipment malfunction/availability, staffing difficulty (unresolved), nursing performance problem, supplies inadequate/inferior, support service/department misunderstanding, communication breakdown, and medical staff–related problem. A brief explanation along with positive suggestions for improvement complete the tool. The problem log is later used to trend such problems after they are identified. This may be maintained manually or by computer and is completed by the manager and reviewed regularly by the staff to monitor problem occurrence and resolution approaches. Spotting trends on (1) shifts, weekends, or holidays, (2) the nature of logged difficulties, (3) resolution effectiveness, and (4) problem recurrence is almost impossible without some type of tracking/trending tool. It is totally unacceptable for today's manager to lack this information, or to try to record it on bits of paper or in his or her head!

Care conferencing is a strategy used in the PI/PR area of the QA umbrella to concurrently or retrospectively review patient care using the group process approach. Conferences commonly study four types of topics: an interesting or unusual patient diagnosis; a deteriorating patient for whom group modification of standards can lead to improved care; selected difficult or challenging behaviors of a patient/patient's significant other, where group process and multidisciplinary input can modify the behavior and/or enhance staff coping abilities; and postmortality or post–Code Blue situations that require group discussion for analysis and critique of care strategies to help improve future care. In all cases, care conference reports are completed to document the event, problems encountered, and improvement resolutions. Care conference reports scanned by the manager over time can often reveal critical trends of problems that often go unnoticed in the day-to-day hassle of unit and department events.

The final activities under this area of the QA umbrella are supervisory rounds for validating staff compliance to standards and interaction with caregivers for problem identification. Four tools are suggested for use by line managers, physician directors/service chiefs, shift leaders, and nursing office supervisors. The supervisory rounds report sheet is designed to document weekly rounds in a clinical area by the first-line and middle manager. It identifies key clinical aspects of care for supervisory observation and columns for recording degree of compliance, cross-referencing results to the caregiver, and writing supportive comments. Open-ended sections contain space for notes related to staff use of protocols and standards of care. The final section is completed at the conclusion of rounds and records: staff learning needs that should be planned for, standards that need to be reviewed with the staff, disciplinary and risk management areas that need immediate attention, and problems that need to be added to the problem log. The tool captures essential information from the rounds, provides the manager with direction for follow-up problem resolution, and provides a quick reference for the next set of rounds in observing for and documenting effectiveness of action taken. Since improvement in performance and care is the essence of QA, this type of tool immediately reflects manager effectiveness because ignoring or simply rerecording unresolved problems is unacceptable (Marker, 1987, pp. 62–63).

Paralleling the supervisory rounds report sheet is the physician rounds report sheet. This tool is completed by the medical director or service chief or someone with the equivalent medical and administrative clout to identify problems of a medical practice nature, pursue corrective action, and hold physicians accountable to a defined level of medical care. Nurse/physician manager rounds should be made on a weekly or bimonthly basis and documented via the rounds tools to provide a regular multidisciplinary look at total systems operation, professional practice, and patient care. These combination rounds do more than just look at the patient: They highlight variables that must be in place to ensure that care can be and is being delivered properly, they identify proper use or abuse of resources, and they demonstrate a joint nursing and medical management effort at mutual problem identification and resolution planning. The physician tool contains sections on the appropriateness of admission diagnosis to the area, appropriate use of consultants, and effective implementation of drug and therapeutic measures. The tool then asks the physician to critique the practitioner's orders; progress notes; use of ancillary and diagnostic services; adequacy of communication with nursing, patient, and family; and discharge orders. Final sections include problem analysis and corrective action planning.

The third PI/PR tool is the unit shift report sheet. This tool is designed for use by the shift leader to track staffing, patient census, and pace/workload of the unit. Open sections are allocated for problem identification in the areas of physician issues, bed utilization, equipment/supplies procurement, and special concerns relative to staff performance. A special box is checked by the shift leader to indicate that additional communication is needed with the unit manager relative to a sensitive staff issue such as potential drug abuse, interpersonal difficulties, failure to complete assignments, substandard performance, and so forth. Finally, a section highlights any incident reports or problem sheets completed on the shift that need to be called to the attention of the manager. This tool is excellent for directing new charge personnel, for making assignments for corrective action, and for tracking effectiveness of actions taken. For example, if QA monitoring determines that a clinical aspect of care such as ventilator management, restraint management, or patient teaching is in noncompliance, the charge nurse can be directed to implement correction plans and report results on the shift report sheet. Information is almost immediately available to the unit manager, allowing the manager to evaluate all components of effectiveness—the plan, the shift leader, and the staff involved.

The final tool for PI/PR is the report sheet used by the nursing office supervisor (NOS). All too frequently, the shift administrative supervisors are not in the mainstream of QA; this tool will focus their energies in assisting with QA on alternate shifts and weekends. The NOS shift report sheet is designed to promote problem identification on off shifts and to extend the monitoring activities of the unit manager into alternate hours. Information collected is primarily generic and directed at compliance with safety and infection control measures, use of protocols and standards of care at the bedside by the nursing staff, and staff compliance to department of nursing structure, process, and outcome standards (Marker, 1989, pp. 47–48).

RELATED COMPONENTS FOR SUCCESSFUL QA

In addition to a practice model that comprehensively organizes a variety of integrated QA activities, five additional components are needed to complete the QA program: a QA plan and calendar, a QA manual, a QA reporting mechanism, a QA committee structure, and an effective QA coordinator.

The QA plan should be written at three levels: hospital, department, and unit. Each plan deals with the 11 elements of a QA plan but is written for a specific level in the organization, beginning with very broad application at the facility level and ending with detailed implications for a clinical area or unit. Table 6-1 lists the elements of a QA plan. Generally the plan is written in an outline, paragraph, narrative style and defines both responsibility and accountability for QA activities. The plan is then translated to a QA calendar, which is posted in a visible area. Events are mapped out for the year so that repeated activities can clearly be seen along with events that take place at periodic intervals. For example, compliance audit topics would be entered in areas of planned structure, process, and outcome review. A minimum of one concurrent monitor topic related to major clinical activities of the area would be posted for each week, along with the responsible staff member. Documentation studies and patient, staff, and physician satisfaction surveys would be plotted, along with the Joint Commission mock survey. Timely continuing education events and credentialing reviews would appear at appropriate times. Additionally, safety and infection control activities would be entered on a quarterly basis. Events that are ongoing, such as active problem identification, incident report tracking, emergency checks, utilization review mechanisms, and preventive maintenance activities, need not be plotted as they occur every month. The QA calendar is visual evidence that QA is systematic, planned, ongoing, and participatively involving all members of the staff (Marker, 1989, p. 50).

The QA manual is the actual record of events taking place. A well-organized manual should be available to the staff on the unit at all times. The unit-based QA manual should sit in a consistent spot next to the unit-based standards manual. Both should be color coded to the clinical service being defined and monitored. The initial section of the QA manual is the QA plan, with the last section devoted to the reporting mechanism. In between are tabs corresponding to the nine elements of the QA umbrella, adjusted for committee structure. Table 6-2 lists the suggested tabs for organizing the QA manual. Every attempt should be made by the QA coordinator and unit manager to create opportunities for the staff to use the manual by entering data in it (shift report sheet, care conference report sheet,

---

Table 6-1 The 11 Elements of a QA Plan

1. organizational pattern of unit/area and scope of clinical activities
2. principles/philosophy of QA
3. objectives of QA plan
4. scope (activities and components)
5. responsibility
6. structure of activities (committees)
7. integration/coordination of activities
8. problem-solving approaches used
9. monitoring activities maintained (10 JCAHO steps)
10. documentation (QA manual and report)
11. evaluation (annual)

Table 6-2 Major Tabs to Organize Content in QA Manual

1. QA plan for service/area
2. annual unit management by objectives
3. unit audit committee
4. unit standards committee
5. continuing education committee
6. credentialing
7. performance appraisal
8. risk management/utilization review committee
9. concurrent monitors
10. active problem identification/ongoing monitors
11. quarterly reports
12. quarterly goal summaries
13. annual QA report

---

individual continuing education record) or reviewing information in it (problem log, unit log, utilization of the unit record, concurrent monitors, audits, preventive maintenance record) (Marker, 1989, pp. 51–52).

The QA reporting mechanism can occur in a variety of ways but its essential components include why, who, when, and what. Reporting occurs to allow managers and staff to share their QA accomplishments, to introspectively take stock of progress, and to integrate lower-level QA activities with departmental and hospital events. The first-line manager supported by the middle manager should be primarily responsible for reporting unit results. The QA coordinator then collates and summarizes these across the department of nursing. The Marker Umbrella Model directs that the QA coordinator also report events across the department on a monthly basis to the nurse executive, either in written or verbal form. Information for this monthly report comes from QA committee meetings and interaction with nurse managers and staff via walking weekly rounds. First-line managers should not have to be bogged down with monthly reports but should submit quarterly unit reports either to the QA coordinator or the middle manager for division collation. The QA coordinator should receive all unit or division quarterly reports and collate them into a quarterly department of nursing QA statement, which is usually then submitted by the department executive to the hospital QA group. Content for the quarterly unit reports should be organized in a simple four-column style addressing data reviewed during the quarter, problems identified or compliance percentages reached, corrective action taken or to be taken, and results obtained. The last column is the most critical and should be expressed in terms of problems eliminated or reduced in frequency or negative impact and increasing standards compliance. Each quarterly unit QA report should be accompanied by the quarterly goal summary, which lists the management by objectives (MBO) goals for the area for the semiannual or annual period and progress made in their accomplishment (completed, in progress, or not yet). The quarterly goal summary validates that managers are goal oriented and that QA has been ultimately successful in accomplishing improvement in systems function, staff performance, and patient care (Marker, 1989, pp. 35–39).

Annual reporting of effectiveness should also be a simple event. The responsibility for compiling the annual report belongs to the QA coordinator. The report should focus on QA results for the year with content coming from quarterly QA reports and other QA sources. The annual summation should not be detailed nor a redundant review of activities conducted. Rather, it should be comprehensive and improvement oriented. The best approach is to briefly summarize department of nursing MBO status with an annual goal summary, similar to the unit tool (MBOs complete, in progress, and not yet complete). Then the report should list the 9 components under the QA umbrella and highlight accomplishments in each area. For example, (1) describe what standards have been developed or revised as a result of QA findings; (2) state the average percent compliance achieved in structure, process, and outcome standards (respectively) as demonstrated by audit and concurrent monitoring; (3) define the number of problems identified via PI/PR tools (in each of the 7 categories if desired) with a breakdown of number of problems resolved and number of problems remaining to be resolved; (4) summarize *UR* results in terms of fiscal stability of the department, overall percentage of time the required staffing component was maintained, staff turnover rate, and success of recruitment/retention efforts; (5) report *RM* results in terms of total incidents filed (with and without significant sequela), compliance to infection control standards, and numbers of significant patient infections (UTI, URI, surgical wound infections, +3 phlebitis), and general safety standards compliance; (6) communicate performance appraisal results via number of nursing personnel promoted, terminated, and given merit/career ladder advances; (7) results from patient, physician, and nursing staff satisfaction surveys; (8) summarize total number of new staff successfully oriented, total number of continuing education programs conducted in direct response to QA findings; (9) summarize number of staff successfully credentialed for special competencies such as ACLS, chemotherapy, fetal monitoring, and so forth. This last issue is a new Joint Commission 1991 requirement in that the nurse executive is expected to report the status of competency of nursing staff to the hospital governing board at least annually (Joint Commission, 1990). Finally, end the report with the percentage of staff and managers actively involved in QA activities across the department.

While all these reportable issues are important and provide the management team with an overall sense of successful QA accomplishment, the four most essential issues remain goal achievement, problem resolution, standards compliance, and staff participation. These four results are synergistically linked. QA is effective if the department of nursing is moving forward with goal achievement. Problems (adverse events, volume indicators, generic screens, occurrences) will be kept below TFE when standards are in consistent compliance (rates of 90 percent or higher) and 75 percent or more of the staff and managers are involved in daily QA activities.

It is essential that the reader comprehend the sequence of events here: Involvement of all staff and managers in QA breeds awareness of standards; awareness of standards increases compliance to standards; compliance to standards prevents and/or controls problematic events. Therefore, the best annual QA report is not a voluminous tome but an organized presentation of accomplishment: annual goal summary of department of nursing MBO status and final analysis of problem resolution, standards compliance, and degree of participative involvement by staff and management (Marker, 1989, pp. 8–9).

Committee structure for QA can also take many forms, but the traditional setup is to have unit representation on the department of nursing QA Committee. The Marker Umbrella Model for QA is less concerned with who is on the committee than with its function. The roles of the QA committee revolve around five responsibilities. The first responsibility includes facilitating QA across the department through educating staff and managers about QA, defining QA mechanisms to be implemented, directing QA events, guiding and supporting activities, and providing feedback on work completed. The second responsibility is coordinating events between central QA committee and decentralized QA unit groups. The third role is standardizing tools, methods, and reporting mechanisms. The fourth function is integrating QA events via linking unit practices with department actions and department events with overall hospital QA measures. The final QA committee responsibility is evaluating overall effectiveness via the annual reporting mechanism (Marker, 1989, pp. 4–6).

Of significant importance are the set up unit-level committees, which must facilitate as much participation as possible by all unit staff. The Umbrella Model suggests that each unit (or clusters of like units if staffing is limited or units are small) create four unit-based committees for QA practice. These committees correspond to the major activities under the umbrella: audit committee, standards committee, continuing education committee, and utilization review/risk management committee. Duties and responsibilities of each committee are listed in the unit QA plan, and each group has a staff or assistant nurse manager chair. All staff sit on one of the committees and may switch groups to obtain a variety of QA experiences. Since participation in QA, standards development, and committee work is part of the unit performance standards, this level of function is a known factor in working on the unit. This wide committee approach is preferred over the traditional unit-based QA committee because using the former approach creates some involvement by all staff, while the traditional committee structure is limited to only a few staff. Remember, it takes maximum staff involvement to create maximum awareness to produce maximum standards compliance and minimal negative events (Marker, 1989, p. 10).

The last related component for a successful QA program is a well-defined QA coordinator role and a highly motivated and competent person in the role. The Umbrella Model suggests that while there are some exceptions in smaller institutions, generally speaking there should be a full-time equivalent devoted to the QA coordinator position in nursing. When this is not the case, it is often a statement by both hospital and nursing administration as to the importance given to QA, and the overall program may suffer due to lack of the strong and consistent leadership that a good QA coordinator can give. Even in departments where size does not allow a full-time coordinator, the same responsibilities assumed by a full-time QA person should be delegated to some managerial nursing position. This, however, will always be less than adequate because priority will have to be given to one position over the other. The 22 roles of the QA coordinator under the Marker Umbrella are outlined in Table 6-3 (Marker, 1989, p. 11).

SEQUENCE OF EVENTS FOR IMPLEMENTATION

In order to implement the Marker Umbrella Model for QA, one must be realistic about one's time frame. QA is like a giant cookie; you can't eat the whole thing in

---

Table 6-3 QA Coordinator Role Areas

1. knowledge base for QA
2. professionalism
3. teaching others
4. self-growth
5. self-validation
6. employee/patient rights
7. safety/risk management
8. legal issues
9. goal setting/participation
10. direction/coordination of others
11. communication
12. working relationships
13. confidentiality
14. problem solving/decision making
15. research
16. planning
17. reporting/evaluation
18. integration/standardization
19. Joint Commission liaison
20. support
21. rounds
22. tracking

one sitting. Take a bite and chew it up; then take another bite, and soon the task is accomplished. It takes 2 to 3 years to develop a comprehensive QA program. Many managers and leaders are both unrealistic and impatient when it comes to developing a sophisticated and effective program. Robotlike, task-oriented, repetitive, paper-oriented activities can be quickly thrown together to satisfy superficial external requirements. But a sophisticated sequence of events carried out by motivated and QA-educated managers with input and full participation by all staff producing measurable and sustained improvement takes time, money, manpower, and tremendous energy! Remember the systems theory: You should get more out of your QA program than you put into it. Otherwise, some significant characteristic is missing.

The development of a sound and effective QA program can be done in five steps if one accepts the dual approach advocated by the Umbrella Model. The dual approach to QA is based on two separate but interdependent series of events: problem identification and resolution and compliance to standards (Marker, 1987, p. 63).

Problem identification and resolution are accomplished through the development and implementation of data sources. Data sources are tools, methods, and mechanisms that are created by the nurse manager for the purpose of data collection and integrated into the daily operation of the unit. Information about unit operation, staff function, and patient care is tracked and trended via these data sources to keep the manager immediately informed about problem occurrences and the effectiveness of resolution interventions. When used consistently, data sources are tools for both problem identification and resolution monitoring. They are extensions of the eyes, ears, and hands of the manager, as they can be in operation 24 hours a day, 7 days a week, 52 weeks a year, while obviously a manager can be physically present only so many hours a day. One third of the nine activities under the Umbrella Model are directed at PI/PR via data sources: utilization review, risk management, and active problem identification/ongoing monitors. These activities are the origin of volume indicators that involve identification, tracking, and trending of adverse events. Many of these data sources were discussed earlier but are again summarized in Table 6-4.

Ensuring compliance with standards comprises the most critical component of the Umbrella Model's activities. Compliance activities are subdivided into two categories: standards development and clinical monitoring. Six of the umbrella's nine activities are directed at compliance to standards mechanisms: four on the left side of the umbrella—standards development, continuing education, credentialing, and performance appraisal—and two on the other side, which are directed at clinical monitoring for compliance to standards: audit and concurrent monitoring. These last two activities are the origin of quality or clinical indicators and, as previously discussed, involve the development of criteria from established standards; calculation of compliance percentages and thresholds; concurrent data col-

Table 6-4 Suggested Partial List of Data Sources for Problem Identification/Resolution

1. satisfaction surveys (patient, staff, physician)
2. generic review questionnaires
3. Joint Commission mock surveys
4. annual continuing education events list
5. continuing education record for individual staff
6. mandatory events attendance list
7. licensure validation tool
8. internal certification record
9. safety/infection control review tool
10. preventive maintenance record
11. incident report tracking form
12. unit log
13. utilization of unit record
14. problem identification sheet
15. problem log
16. care conference report sheets
17. report sheets (supervisory, physician, NOS, shift leader)

lection, tabulation, and analysis; corrective action planning, and follow-up monitoring. Table 6-5 reviews the activities under the dual approach.

With the understanding of the dual approach and the purpose of the nine Umbrella components, it is now appropriate to spell out the five steps for developing a QA program. First, complete the related components for success: QA plan, calendar, manual, reporting mechanism, central and unit committee structure, and QA coordinator position and role description. Second, implement the three PI/PR focus activities by developing the necessary data sources (see Table 6-4). Third, devote concentrated time at developing structure, process, and outcome standards at the generic department and unit-based levels (see Figure 6-1). Fourth, heavily focus on compliance to standards monitoring. Fifth,

Table 6-5 Dual Approach Activities under Marker Umbrella Model for QA

Active PI/PR Focus	Compliance to Standards Focus
1. Utilization review	1. Standards development
2. Risk management	2. Continuing education
3. Active PI/PR via ongoing data sources	3. Credentialing
	4. Performance appraisal
	5. Audit
	6. Concurrent monitoring

implement staff development, credentialing and performance appraisal systems to support all QA activities (Table 6-6).

APPLICATION OF UMBRELLA MODEL TO OTHER DEPARTMENTS

The Marker Umbrella Model for QA is universally applicable to all departments within the health care organization. The major points of the QA plan, manual, and reporting mechanism are transferrable to every service. The major themes of PI/ PR and compliance to standards are essential to all direct and indirect patient care areas. Since all managers are responsible for minimizing problems that interfere with effective department function and goal attainment, the data sources outlined may be used across the board with modification to the service. Since all managers and personnel are expected to function in concert with standards, all that is required in most departments is to expand their traditional "policy/procedure" thinking into standards development. Then it is a natural evolution to spend QA energy increasing compliance to the standards so that problem occurrences will be minimized. It is the responsibility of the hospital QA coordinator to assist each department head in the development of the area's QA plan, data sources, and standards. The QA coordinator can work with each department head to take one Umbrella activity at a time and define its application to the area. For example, risk management is a universal mechanism of QA. How does one define risk in the pharmacy? Precisely what actions are necessary to reduce these risks? What data sources could be designed to monitor these risks and document that they are under control? Similar thought processes would take place in all departments in relation to each component of the Umbrella.

CLINICAL IMPACT

The clinical impact of the Marker Umbrella Model for QA can best be realized when it is implemented fully and in concert with the sister model for standards development. Six measurable results can be achieved using the QA Umbrella approach. First, staff accountability to standards increases through standards development, awareness, and involvement in compliance monitoring. Increased accountability means a higher degree of professionalism and consistency of performance by staff and improved patient care both in process and in outcome.

Second, documentation of standards compliance and effectiveness leads to validation of the standards or modification of content. Thus there is a built-in mechanism for constant review and revision of standards content through the QA process.

Table 6-6 Five Sequential Steps for Developing a QA Program

Steps	Marker QA Umbrella Model Tools
1. Complete related components.	Plan and calendar Manual Reporting tools/mechanism Central/unit committee structure
2. Implement 3 PI/PR focused activities via data sources for UR, RM, and API.	Unit log tracking tool Utilization of unit trending tool Safety/infection control reviews Emergency equipment checks Preventive maintenance checks Incident report tracking Problem identification sheets Problem/resolution trending log Patient care conferencing tool Supervisor rounds sheet (nursing) Supervisor rounds sheet (physician)
3. Develop comprehensive and sophisticated standards at the department and unit level related to structure, process, and outcome.	Generic and unit specific structure Job descriptions/performance standards Generic/unit specific procedures Generic/unit specific protocols Generic/unit specific forms and guidelines Unit specific standards of care
4. Initiate consistent compliance monitoring via quality indicators/criteria development evolving from predefined standards.	Criteria development sheets Data retrieval forms
5. Create integrated systems of continuing education, staff competency credentialing, and recognition/reward to support all QA activities.	Continuing education events list Individual staff education/professional accomplishment record Mandatory events record Licensure validation record Internal certification record Clinical privilege approval record Performance appraisal tools

Third, the Umbrella forces a comprehensive and integrated view of QA and brings managerial responsibilities in line with the staff clinical responsibilities for QA. QA is no longer seen as isolated and redundant paper work but a viable vehicle for making things better. All aspects of systems function, staff performance, and patient care are examined. Structure, process, and outcome all receive equal attention, with the understanding that while outcomes are the ultimate measurement of the worth of the care and caregiver, consistent structure and well-executed process are the roads to positive patient outcomes.

Fourth, the roles of the manager and staff for QA are clarified. The Umbrella Model doesn't just focus on the process of QA, as so many articles and conferences do. It teaches the activities of QA and delineates what managers and staff alike should do to implement each activity. Leaders learn to manage through quality assurance activities, not just go through the motions in an attempt to satisfy external requirements. Managers learn to be creative in the development and implementation of data sources and equally creative in problem resolution approaches, with a full awareness of the responsibility they bear for effectiveness. Staff learn that QA is not a mysterious phenomenon but a strategy for expanding their responsibilities for evaluation of care. Staff get excited about being involved in activities that produce results instead of meaningless paper and statistics. The umbrella's committee structure, approach to spot checking via concurrent monitoring, tools for active problem identification, cross-referencing of QA results with caregiver names, professional credentialing mechanisms, and linkage of QA results with performance appraisal are but a few ways that QA influences staff function and feedback.

Fifth, the model's concrete tools and predesigned forms, especially those for criteria development and data retrieval, teach managers and staff the art of sophisticated criteria writing and the technique of establishing compliance goals, analyzing data, and developing corrective action plans. These are all critical skills that are commonly poorly developed in many QA programs.

Sixth, and finally, because the umbrella is universally applicable, it can produce like results that can be used to compare effectiveness across departments of nursing. Without this comparability, the real essence of QA is lost: What is the best way to operate a nursing system? What is safe staff performance? What is effective patient care? And what is appropriate QA?

REFERENCES

Joint Commission on Accreditation of Healthcare Organizations. (1986). *Quality Review Bulletin*: Special Publication.

Joint Commission on Accreditation of Healthcare Organizations. (1990). *Accreditation Manual for Hospitals* (Vol. II: Scoring guidelines. Nursing care. NC2), 18.

Marker, C.G.S. (1987). The Marker Umbrella Model for quality assurance: Monitoring and evaluating professional practice. *Journal of Nursing Quality Assurance, 1*, 52–63.

Marker, C.G.S. (1988a). Practical tools for QA: Criteria development sheet and data retrieval form. *Journal of Nursing Quality Assurance, 2*, 43–54.

Marker, C.G.S. (1988b). *Setting standards for professional nursing*. Philadelphia: CV Mosby.

Marker, C.G.S. (1989). The Marker Umbrella Model for quality assurance. Unpublished handouts for workshop, Marker Systems, Severna Park, Maryland.

7

The Pyramid for Nursing Quality Assurance

P. Mardeen Atkins, BSN, RN, Nursing Quality Management Coordinator, *Cleveland Clinic Foundation, Cleveland, Ohio.*

Deborah M. Nadzam, PhD, RN, Project Manager, Indicator Development, *Joint Commission on Accreditation of Healthcare Organizations, and Former Director of Nursing Research, Cleveland Clinic Foundation, Cleveland, Ohio*

Cathy M. Ceccio, MSN, RN, Former Director Orthopedics/Neuroscience *Nursing, Cleveland Clinic Foundation, Cleveland, Ohio.*

In the past several years, there have been major changes in the health care environment. These changes reflect the public's increasing concern with the quality of health care and payers' concern with the increasing costs of that care. Health care institutions are being asked to demonstrate that they can provide quality care while still controlling the costs. There is also increasing emphasis on quality of care by regulatory agencies, such that quality assurance (QA) activities have become a priority in health care institutions.

The Division of Nursing at the Cleveland Clinic Foundation is comprised of 2000 employees working in 37 specialty units/areas. These units/areas are divided into five clinical departments: surgical/oncology, medical, cardiothoracic, critical care, and operating room. Designing a QA program within the Division of Nursing that would meet all the external and internal needs of these departments was indeed a challenge. This chapter describes the development, implementation, and utilization of the model that was eventually developed, the Pyramid for Nursing Quality Assurance (PQA).

THEORETICAL BASIS OF PQA

Designing and then implementing such a comprehensive program for QA required identification of its theoretical underpinnings. Two significant areas reviewed in this process were QA/control and organizational/management theory.

The Joint Commission's Impact on Quality of Care Program Development

The Joint Commission on Accreditation of Healthcare Organizations (Joint Commission) has been a leader in the promotion of quality health care since its

81

establishment in 1951. At the time of the original development of the PQA, the Joint Commission's standards for QA called for the existence of a program that monitors compliance to standards of care and/or practice. The monitoring activities were to be planned, with demonstrated follow-up action when indicated and subsequent evaluation of the effect of that action. In 1986 the Joint Commission introduced plans for its Agenda for Change, which included description of a nine-step process for monitoring and evaluation (Joint Commission, 1986). In 1987 the process was revised to include setting thresholds for evaluation. The thresholds are to guide the organization in taking action to improving quality. In addition, the Agenda for Change proposed paying increased attention to monitoring patient outcomes.

Juran's and Deming's Influence on Quality Control

Taking the lead from industry's recent interest in continuous improvement and statistical process control, the writings of Joseph M. Juran and W. Edwards Deming were reviewed for their relevance to nursing practice. Both Juran and Deming emphasized the need for management to promote and support continuous improvement.

The Juran Trilogy details the three universal processes of managing quality: quality planning, quality control, and quality improvement. The initial activity, planning, calls for identification of customers and their needs, with subsequent development of product and process designs. The second activity is control, that is, correcting defects, preventing things from getting worse, and putting out fires. The third step is improvement, or recognizing opportunities to further improve quality. By improvement Juran means "the organized creation of beneficial change; the attainment of unprecedented levels of performance." (Juran, 1989). He emphasizes upper management's involvement in the processes of managing quality, from identifying quality goals to participating in specific projects.

W. Edwards Deming also underscores the importance of management direction and participation in quality improvement activities (Walton, 1986). He details 14 points to support continuous improvement and 7 deadly diseases that impede improvement. The 14 points are all directives to management improving communication within the organization, breaking down barriers to participation, and enhancing employee moral and performance. The 7 deadly diseases relate to an organization's shortsightedness, excessive costs, and ineffective employee performance review practices. Deming is a proponent of statistical process control; he advocates basing decisions on accurate and timely data. Statistical methods can be used to understand variance and set acceptable upper and lower control limits to that variance (Deming, 1982).

Contingency Management Theory

Synthesizing the influence of the Joint Commission, Juran, and Deming, it is apparent that the emphasis of quality monitoring activities has evolved from assessment of quality (planning), to assurance of quality (control), and now to ongoing monitoring and improvement of quality. It was important that the new program for the authors' hospital QA incorporate these current trends.

A review of the literature on organizational and management theory was conducted, and of the theories surveyed, contingency management theory seemed to offer an approach that would support the principles of quality improvement. Contingency management theory views an organization as an open system interacting with its environment to maintain stability. Leadership style and action are contingent upon the situation and the work to be done. Charns and Schaefer (1983) conceptualize a contingency model for management of a health care organization that includes six elements: environment, purposes and goals, work, structure, coordination, and people.

According to Charns and Schaefer, environment includes everything outside the organization. In health care it encompasses patients and their families, competitors, students, regulating boards, government, insurance companies, and the surrounding community.

Purposes and goals are primary to an organization. Purpose is the reason for its existence; goals or objectives are the targets of its direct work. A health care organization's purpose is to provide services to patients. Goals and objectives vary somewhat by organization.

Work is the central focus of the organizational model, defined in general as "energy directed at bringing about a change in the state of something " (p. 81). Work is positioned between the organization's purposes and other elements. Three types of work are described by contingency theory: direct, management, and support. Direct work is driven by the purposes and goals of the organization. It is the most task oriented and most obviously patient outcome–oriented. Management work focuses on the interface of the organization and the environment and on maintaining balance among the other elements. Management work facilitates direct work. Support work is driven by direct and management work more so than by the organization's purposes and goals.

Structure refers to the division of work and assignment of responsibilities and authority. The organizational structure, reporting relationships, and job descriptions are examples of structure.

Coordination can be viewed as the mechanism for achieving optimum performance. It may include coordinating between or within elements.

People within the organization constitute the crucial element most needing understanding and managing. Both individuals and groups of people interact with the environment and within the structure of the organization, working to accomplish purposes and goals.

Contingency management theory, coupled with the current trends in the monitoring of quality of care, provided the building blocks for our new QA program. The inclusion of the elements of contingency management theory, ongoing improvement, and management involvement were recognized as desirable objectives of the program.

BUILDING THE PYRAMID FOR QA

To create the new QA program based on QA trends and contingency management theory, it was first necessary to be able to visualize the model.

The Five Basic Objectives

In the effort to redefine the QA program for nursing at the Cleveland Clinic Foundation, five objectives were set (numbered below). The program needed to (1) *support the primary mission of the Division of Nursing* (to deliver high-quality professional care to patients) and (2) *include as many nurses as possible*. Based on the belief that each position in the Division contributes to patient care in some way, the program needed to also (3) *monitor the quality of manager's work, as well as that of direct caregivers*. Finally, the program needed to (4) *be easily implemented and maintained* and (5) *meet the standards for QA established by the Joint Commission*.

All five elements of contingency management theory were included in the new model. The five objectives set to redefine the QA program became the premises on which the model was based:

1. The ultimate goal of all nursing employees is to deliver the highest possible quality of care to the patients.
2. The work of all nursing employees is driven by the four missions (purposes) of the Division of Nursing: (a) provide the highest quality professional nursing care, (b) participate in nursing research, (c) provide education to staff and patients, and (d) serve as a resource to the community.
3. The work of the Division of Nursing is divided into three kinds: direct (hands-on), support (environment, systems), and management (decision making).
4. The work of the Division of Nursing occurs within a structure of four levels: individual, unit, department (groupings of similar units), and division (all areas and personnel within nursing).

5. Improving quality is accomplished through ongoing monitoring and evaluation of performance.

Visual Representation of the Model

To clarify the model, the five premises were depicted as three nested pyramidals, prompting the name "Pyramid for Quality Assurance" (Nadzam & Atkins, 1987) (see Figure 7-1). The three pyramids represent the three types of work (direct, support, and management); the four levels intersecting them are

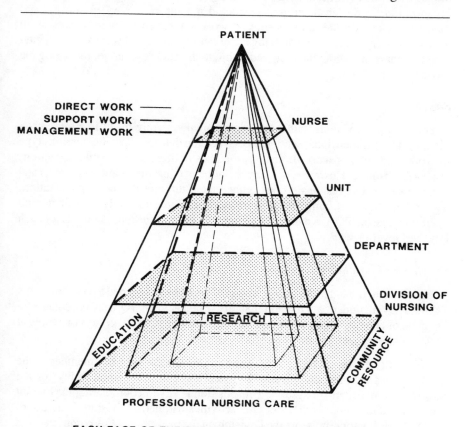

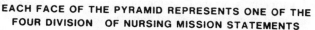

Figure 7-1 Cleveland Clinic Foundation Division of Hospital Nursing Pyramid for Quality Assurance.
Source: Courtesy of the Cleveland Clinic Foundation, Division of Hospital Nursing, Cleveland, OH.

related to organizational structure (individual, unit, department, and division); each side of the four-sided figure symbolizes a mission statement. The focus of all work is the patient, positioned at the top of the pyramid. The work of quality improvement has a sound base—the entire Division of Nursing, supported by ancillary services (middle pyramid) and enveloped by management, the outermost pyramid.

Types of Work

Direct work is performed by caregivers and is at the core of health care service. Support work is performed by persons who provide services to others within the organization; in this instance we considered nursing resource departments and indirect workers on the units as support work. Management work occurs at all levels: the individual nurse managing his or her own time and work with patients, the head nurse managing the unit, and so on, to the nurse executive, managing the Division as a whole.

Structure

The multiple divisions within the tripyramidal structure result in a total of 48 different three-dimensional sections. Each section defines a specific mission, type of work, and level of work. In reality, the lines of demarcation between sections are not so absolute. However, primary assignment of problems and/or projects and major areas of QA responsibilities is facilitated through this conceptualization. Two other structural components were necessary to effectively coordinate and operationalize the PQA: a data management system and specific standards for each type and level of work.

People and Coordination

Finally, specific individuals and groups of people were needed to coordinate the PQA. They included a Division Quality Management (QM) Coordinator, a Division of Nursing Quality Management Committee (QMC), groups of people at each work level, and information specialists.

Division QM Coordinator. The Division QM Coordinator is a member of the QMC, serves as a resource to the Division, and assumes responsibility for the information management system. This position is key to coordinating the overall program and in a sense orchestrates the activities within the Division. In addition, the QM coordinator represents the Division on the institution's QA committee and serves as a liaison to other divisions and departments.

Quality Management Committee (QMC). The QMC is a standing committee reporting to the chair of the Division of Nursing. Membership is specifically defined to allow for representation from all of the pyramid sections. One committee member may represent more than one of the 48 sections. For example, the Nursing Education Coordinator represents support work and management work at the department level, and the mission to educate caregivers. Thus an 18-member committee can adequately represent the 48 subsections. The resulting multilevel representation on the committee provides the committee with a perspective of the work from each type, level, and mission.

Other Departmental and Unit Committees. Groups of persons within the several departments and units actually perform the monitoring and evaluation activities, realizing the process of unit-based QA. Formation of the groups is left to the direction of unit and departmental manager, although each unit is asked to name a registered nurse, preferably in a staff nurse position, to serve as the unit QA coordinator.

Information Specialists. Information specialists are essential to plan for the effective and efficient handling of the volume of data generated by the PQA. Assistance from the Division's information resource manager is sought in this regard.

Initiation of the Program

Following administrative approval of the PQA, the QMC was formed. Specific individuals were asked to represent related types, levels, and missions of work. The PQA was then presented to the newly formed committee. The primary responsibilities of the QMC were delineated: to oversee the development, implementation, and maintenance of the PQA and to educate the staff about it. To operationalize the PQA, the QMC first offered educational programs about QA and the PQA.

Education played a major role in the implementation and maintenance of the PQA program. At the outset, a Division-wide survey assessed nurses' experience with and understanding of QA and identified current unit QA practices. Using this information the QMC planned a 1-day workshop for all managers and unit QA coordinators. The presentation focused on the PQA framework, the Joint Commission's 10-step monitoring and evaluation (M & E) model, the meaning of "unit-based QA program," and the development and/or refinement of standards.

Follow-up sessions to the workshop were offered to individual units or groups. These sessions focused only on the QA process: defining the scope of care, identifying important aspects of care, and identifying indicators for monitoring and evaluation purposes. The sessions were informal, usually conducted on the units, and focused on the unit's education needs related to the M & E process. These sessions proved very beneficial as the staff felt more comfortable asking questions and expressing their ideas in small groups. It was also easier to use these meetings to plan the unit's M & E activities.

FINE TUNING THE PROGRAM

The results of the initial steps taken to operationalize the PQA included a heightened awareness about QA and about the expectations that the new program would drive the initiative to improve quality of care in the Division of Nursing. After several unit meetings, it became apparent that by focusing only on the M & E process without relating it to the PQA model was leading the staff to think of them as two unrelated programs. Some revisions were needed in our approach. Three target areas were identified: (1) provision of additional educational programs, (2) provision of additional structure to QA committees, and (3) development of an information management system.

Additional Educational Programs

The follow-up sessions were somewhat successful in educating the staff about QA; however, they did not help the staff understand the connection between the PQA and the QA process. The staff perceived the PQA model as complicated and unrelated to their everyday practice. It was also apparent that the managers and unit QA coordinators needed additional coaching to feel more confident with their roles as coordinators. Finally, the need for an educational program for the orientation of new staff, graduate nurses, registered nurses, and the like, was identified.

Revamping the Follow-Up Sessions

Revamping the follow-up sessions took priority over orientation sessions, to ensure that managers and unit QA coordinators were knowledgeable and comfortable with the program objectives. The sessions were formalized to demonstrate the relationship between the Joint Commission's 10-step M & E model and the PQA. These sessions were offered to one clinical department (group of similar units) at a time and were presented to the unit QA coordinators, the unit management staff, and director of the department. Each of the 10 steps was described. The following highlights of the revised follow-up sessions demonstrate approaches used to relate the 10-step M & E model to the PQA.

Scope of Care. In the initial workshop, the unit QA coordinators had identified their scope of care: the patient population, major diagnoses, treatments provided, the providers of those treatments, and where these treatments are provided. In the follow-up sessions, the scope of care was written and placed into the unit QA manuals. This helped the units be more focused when identifying the important aspects of care and the corresponding indicators. To present a complete picture of the unit, the skill mix of caregivers and type of care delivery system for the unit were included in the written scope of care.

At this point, a scope of care was also written for the Division, with input from the QMC and the Nursing Executive Council. Several of the clinical departments also identified the scope of care for their common patient population. Defining the scopes of care for the different levels of work within the Division has helped make the PQA model more functional for the staff by demonstrating that each level performs various degrees of the three types of work.

Important Aspects of Care. The important aspects of care are the major clinical functions that occur on the unit, with a focus on those that are high volume, high risk, or problem prone for patient or staff. For monitoring and evaluation activities across the Division, six aspects of care were identified: (1) use of the nursing process, (2) patient education, (3) adequacy of discharge planning, (4) patient safety, (5) medication administration, and (6) intravenous therapy. Following the units' identification of their respective aspects of care, the Division then selected the most repeatedly identified apsects of care and established them as Division-level aspects in addition to the six above. In all, there were over 30 aspects of care identified for monitoring and evaluation activities.

Establishing the data collection and information processing of these many aspects became cumbersome and difficult to manage. To more effectively deal with data and information gleaned from M & E activities, the definition of "aspect of care" was broadened at the Division level. Five general categories for aspects were defined: (1) discharge planning, (2) nursing process, (3) patient education, (4) patient safety, and (5) patient satisfaction. The units then specified the focus of each aspect of care on their level. For example, a Division-level aspect of care is patient safety; within this category one unit may choose to focus on patient falls, while another focuses on medication administration. In addition to streamlining the collection and analysis step, this strategy helped the staff convert the PQA into practice.

Although the emphasis of identifying aspects of care was primarily on clinical functions (direct work), there were aspects identified for support work and management work. Blood glucose meter maintenance and compliance with regulatory agency standards were noted to be important aspects of support work. Timely conduction of performance evaluations and efficient resource utilization were aspects of management work.

Indicators. Indicators, the measurable variables that focus on structure, process, or outcome of care, are used to collect data about important aspects of care. The indicators can be derived from literature, standards, specialty organizations, or staff expertise. Initially, indicators and standards were treated separately. Indicators were set to measure the standard of care. This was confusing to the staff, as in many cases the standard was simply being rewritten as an indicator. To eliminate this confusion, "indicator" was substituted for the word "standard" when developing a monitoring activity. The data were collected on measurable elements that reflected process or outcome. For example, here are the indicators and measurable elements for the patient safety category of the intravenous therapy aspect of care:

Aspect of care:
Patient safety—intravenous therapy
Indicators:
(1) Policies and procedures for intravenous therapy will be followed (process).
(2) Patient will have intravenous therapy without complications (outcome).
Measurable elements:
(1) Tubing changed every 72 hours.
(2) Site rotation every 72 hours.
(3) Dressing changed every 72 hours.
(4) Bottle/bag changed every 24 hours.
(5) No sign of complication at site.

This strategy resulted in easier presentation to staff and increased staff understanding due to their improved ability to separate the monitoring activity from the standardized care plans and protocols.

Threshold for Evaluation. The fifth step in the M & E model—establishing a threshold for evaluation (the point at which intensive evaluation of the data takes place)—was the most problematic for the staff. It was difficult to understand how to set the threshold and what it meant when you reached the threshold. The strategy used to help the staff with this step was to present the threshold for evaluation as the point for action—the point at which you can no longer let the problem continue without developing a plan of action to correct it. This approach also minimized the tendency to set extreme thresholds.

The QMC and the Nursing Executive Council set the thresholds for evaluation for the division-level indicators. These are re-evaluated and raised on an annual basis. The units then set their own thresholds for evaluation, with the expectation that they would be at least at the level of the division threshold.

Data Collection and Analysis. Data are collected for each indicator on an ongoing basis. Existing data sources were identified, and their use was strongly encouraged. The data provide a performance score for each indicator that can be compared to the threshold for evaluation. Data sources within the Division included the Medicus Corporation's Nursing Productivity NPAQ and Quality Management System (NPAQ-QM), the patient classification system, the incident reporting system, and the performance management system. (These systems are described in detail below.)

The staff easily understood data collection processes, as they were very accustomed to this activity through the NPAQ-QM system and the reporting of unusual events via the incident reporting system. There was a greater problem with how to use the information processed from the data. The units were being overwhelmed with data and information and were having difficulty organizing and prioritizing it for analysis.

The education efforts were directed at organizing and analyzing the data and developing a plan of action if the threshold for evaluation was reached. An exercise was developed around the intravenous therapy aspect of care. The groups were asked to determine if the threshold for evaluation had been reached, and if so, what additional data were needed for further evaluation. Actual scores were used for each department so that by the end of a department-level analysis, a plan of action was developed for the common problem areas across the department. This exercise was presented at department meetings for two quarters to ensure that the staff were comfortable with data analysis. Another benefit of this educational strategy was that it demonstrated the interaction of the different levels of work and types of work, helping to operationalize the PQA.

The revision of follow-up educational sessions for the managers, unit QA coordinators, and unit staff proved to strengthen the connection between the PQA and the QA process. Nurses throughout the Division began contributing to the operationalization of the PQA and, more important, to the continual improvement of the quality of nursing care provided to patients.

Orientation and Continuing Education

In addition to revamping the follow-up sessions, educational programs were planned for the orientation of new staff and other staff on the units who had not participated in earlier programs. Two methods were used: videotapes and computer-assisted instruction.

A videotape describing the PQA, the 10-step M & E model, and how the two relate was prepared and used in the 4th week of the orientation for graduate nurses and registered nurses. At the end of the videotape, the orientees participated in an exercise on developing a monitoring activity. The intravenous therapy example was again used, but the group had to determine the elements to be measured, how the data were to be collected, and who would do the analysis. Scores from the Division level were distributed, and the group then analyzed the data. The emphasis was on the first steps of the monitoring and evaluation process, rather than on the data analysis and reporting steps.

As a supplement to the videotape and a method to reinforce the education to other staff, computer-assisted instruction was utilized. This program briefly explained the model and the 10-step M & E process, relating each step to employees' units. This has been very successful and will eventually replace the videotape session.

We found that education has provided a vital link to the success of our QA program. We too are practicing continuous improvement by constantly evaluating the effectiveness of our educational approach and revising it as necessary.

QA Committees

The QA committees on all three levels were in need of additional structure. Membership and functions were reviewed.

Division QMC

The Division QMC had representation from all sections of the PQA. Initially, the focus of the committee had been twofold: to oversee the structure during implementation and to educate the staff. In order to fine tune and then maintain the QA program, the focus of the committee changed. The QMC began to focus on improvement through peer and practice review. The QMC began to review divisional data to determine the ownership of newly identified areas in need of improvement and to identify issues at the unit and/or departmental levels that might be more appropriately addressed at the divisional level.

Given the change in focus, the need for input from the unit QA coordinators was recognized. Each department named one unit QA coordinator to serve on the QMC. The change in membership did result in greater input from the staff nurse level, strengthening commitment to the unit-based QA philosophy. The staff nurses on the QMC also began to attend their department's management meetings at least quarterly; these meetings are devoted to QA. This has ensured a strong communication link among all levels.

Department-Level Committees

Each of the departments within the Division had regularly scheduled meetings that included the director of the department, the unit management staff, and clinical instructors. These meetings became the forum for departmental QA activities. On a quarterly basis, the entire agenda is devoted to QA. The unit QA coordinators for the department and the Division QA coordinator are present at these meetings.

The broad agenda items for these meetings include (1) discussion of results of M & E activities occurring within the department, (2) planning of future M & E activities, (3) sharing of activities or ideas occurring on the units, (4) discussion of any issues or problems units are having with the QA process, (5) communication of changes in the Division's QA activities and/or program, and (6) provision of information concerning external environment issues related to reimbursement and quality of care. The group is also responsible for the department's development and/or revision of standards of care, performance, and management; development of indicators; and annual review of the "Suggested Plans of Care" for their patient population.

Department-level QA committees had not been started when the PQA was implemented. This resulted in a weak link in the lines of communication about QA activities and did not help to promote the inter-relationship between the different types of work at the different levels. Since the implementation of the department level QA meetings, many of the communication problems have been resolved. By using an existing meeting group, additional time was not spent in meetings. It has promoted many joint projects between units within the department and has lead to the resolution of some common problems across departments.

Unit-Level Committees

The QA committees at the unit level are the most important of the structure. If there is not buy-in and participation at this level, then any QA structure will be ineffective.

The structure and function of the unit QA committee is determined by the unit. Suggestions for involving staff in different monitoring and evaluation activities and for educating the staff about the QA program were presented at the initial educational workshop. The unit's responsibilities were (1) identification of the important aspects of care and corresponding indicators, (2) collection and analysis of data, (3) reporting of results, (4) planning and acting to affect change when indicated, (5) evaluation of the effectiveness of the action, and (6) education of staff about the QA process.

The hardest barrier to overcome was convincing the units that they did have the final say in what they would do for QA. There would be support and consultative assistance provided, but they were responsible for the program's impact on the unit.

The units with the most effective programs are those that have a committee comprised of 2 to 3 staff nurses, with input from the clinical instructor. Each member of the committee is responsible for a different aspect of care, involving other members of the unit staff in the designing of the activity, data collection, and data analysis. The results of the monitoring are then presented at the unit staff meetings, with discussions of the findings and determination of whether further action is necessary. It is important that all members of the unit staff feel a sense of responsibility for the quality of care delivered on the unit. This has been accomplished through the involvement of all staff in the M & E process. QA on these units is not viewed as a meaningless paper exercise that is done simply to be in compliance with the Joint Commission. On the contrary, the staff view the program and activities as a vehicle for effecting change and improvement.

Information Management System

A unit-based QA program in a large institution can generate an abundance of data that could easily be lost or duplicated if an effective information management system is not developed. Even before the implementation of the PQA, the need for a computerized information management system was anticipated.

The four main database systems used to monitor the quality of nursing care are maintained within the Division of Nursing: (1) the NPAQ-QM, (2) the NPAQ patient classification system, (3) the incident reporting system, and (4) the performance management system. Each of these database systems is briefly described, followed by a discussion of the integration of them through an information management system for quality.

Medicus Quality Management System

The NPAQ-QM is used as the primary data collection tool, providing consistency in both the development of indicators and measurable elements and the scoring process. Many of the measurable elements identified by the units are included as standard NPAQ-QM data elements, thus already providing data collection and analysis capabilities. The customization functions of the NPAQ-QM allowed for entry of additional measurable elements into the system. Thus data collection and analysis for very specific unit activities were facilitated through this software. The NPAQ-QM system generates monthly and trend reports on major objective categories, as well as subobjective categories and specific indicators. There is no mechanism at this time allowing for the introduction of threshold values, which would enable a "signaling" to occur if the threshold is reached.

Other Systems

Other databases available to nursing include the occupational injury system, the infection control system, and financial systems. Some of these systems provide regular reports to nursing; others generate reports as requested.

Integration of Data and Information

An information management system integrating data from the above systems is still under development. The function of this system will be to pull data and information from all the existing data sources and to provide comprehensive reports reflecting the activities and effectiveness of the QA program. The system will be personal computer (PC)-based, but the managers have access to the information through either networking or report distribution.

The information management system is only part of data management. The staff who use the system have to understand what the system is, what it can do, and what they need to do to make the system effective. The data collection forms must be easily understood and developed with checks to ensure that all the data are complete. The staff also need to know what information is available so that they can decide what they need.

Information reports must be easily understood, too. Sending out all available data becomes overwhelming to the staff. Presenting information and data in the form of a graph or chart enables the staff to visualize the progress they have made, as well as identify areas still in need of improvement. More detailed data can be provided when a threshold for evaluation is reached, or when the staff request it for other purposes (e.g., more formal study of variables).

Patient Classification and Staffing System

A second Medicus product, the NPAQ patient classification and staffing modules, has been in place since 1985. Data from this system have been particularly useful in monitoring management work as it relates to resource utilization. The data have also been used to analyze trends related to unusual events (e.g., are medication-related events a function of staffing numbers?). At this time, classification and staffing data are manually entered into the incident reporting system to facilitate this analysis.

Incident Reporting System

A paper system for reporting unusual events had been in existence for a long time in the Division. The system was automated in 1986 and then completely reconfigured following the implementation of the PQA. It is now a stand-alone PC system, programmed using d-Base and Clipper. The report form used by staff is a paper version of the computer screen, facilitating data entry. The system is able to provide detailed reports about a single event or describe trends in events for a unit or department or for the Division. Data from the acuity system have been added, which allows the tracking of trends related to resources. The system was also developed to interface with other databases in order to provide a more complete picture of influences on quality of care (i.e., the occupational injury system).

Management System

ouse developed system is the performance management system. atabase used to track the management aspect of work related to timely conduction of performance appraisals. It is programmed similarly to the incident reporting system, producing numerical and graphic reports on both monthly and cumulative levels. This information has been particularly helpful to directors and the chair of the Division when managers' performance is being evaluated.

UTILIZING THE PYRAMID FOR QA

The primary use of the PQA program has been to improve the quality of care. The success of the program is primarily a result of acceptance and support for the program at the Division's administrative level. This support, coupled with the use of the PQA as a framework for assessing both the environment in which nursing is practiced and the delivery of care system, has led to improvement in patient care and staff's increased awareness about and appreciation for QA activities.

Acceptance and Support of the Program

The success of the PQA is primarily due to the support for the program at the administrative level. There has been support from this level since the origin of the PQA. The directors of nursing have been actively involved in the QMC and have participated in the education programs. In addition, all new programs, patient related or operational, now have a monitoring and evaluation component built into them. Further evidence of administrative support is seen in the use of the PQA to develop a framework for changing nursing practice at the Cleveland Clinic Foundation (CCF).

Assessment of the Environment and Delivery of Care System

The PQA was used as the framework for assessing the factors internal and external to the Division of Nursing that influence quality of care. An understanding of the current environment is an essential step to planned change. The PQA was selected as the organizational framework to study the environment because of the staff's familiarity with its concepts. In addition, the model helps to communicate the institution's overall commitment to excellence in patient care and integrates the three types of work, on four levels, according to the four missi

The assessment of factors included the parameters of nurse-to-p
nurse, nurse-to-physician, and nurse-to-environment interaction
assessment, the PQA served as a useful model for identifying
interdependency of those providing direct patient care and t

support and management positions was clearly seen. Although many changes can be made at the level of the individual nurse or unit to improve patient outcomes, our assessment of related factors indicated that many changes must be collaboratively planned, implemented, and evaluated. Thus the PQA emphasized the role of all disciplines in direct, support, and management work to affect change and continuously improve the quality of care.

The PQA was also used in this way on the department and unit levels. For example, staff on two units were concerned about their ability to help patients feel prepared for discharge. Both of these units care for patients undergoing major joint replacements and other complex orthopaedic procedures and thus place a high priority on the divisional standard for adequacy of discharge planning. Simultaneously, the institution had restated its commitment to establishing discharge plans for each service. Multidisciplinary discharge rounds were established, reflecting the integrated role of nurses in direct care, support work, and management work. The multidisciplinary approach also illustrated the mutual dependence of the nursing staff on physicians, social workers, and physical and occupational therapists to formulate or complete their part of the plan. At the same time, unit-and/or specialty-specific job expectations emphasized the value and importance of discharge planning. Monitoring activities for effectiveness of discharge planning would then be structured around patient satisfaction with discharge planning, with incorporation of results into performance appraisal.

The assessment of factors influencing nursing practice helped to evaluate the delivery of care system. The inner core of the pyramid exemplifies the importance of clinical practice to optimal patient outcomes. The practice of the individual nurse at the bedside is influenced by the professional organizational values of colleagues from the unit, clinical department, and Division. Support and management work can also influence the execution of the nurse's clinical practice. Educational opportunities, system supports, and management coaching and guidance all help to create a milieu in which nursing practice can flourish. Often, the nursing unit has the greatest impact on the professional's normative clinical practice, so it is reasonable to believe that unit-based QA activities have a significant opportunity for effecting changes in clinical practice. Changes in support systems, management approaches, and the role of the nurse are occurring as a result of evaluating factors and delivery of care.

Noted Areas of Improvement in Patient Care

onal level, the decrease in the number of patient falls and the *Performan..* venous therapy problems have been the most noticeable areas of

Another in- ugh the tracking of the types of falls, the ages of the patients, This is a small falls, units with high-risk patients were able to develop and implement interventions for their patient populations. These interventions were shared with other units and were tailored to fit their patient populations. Through another Division-wide activity, the monitoring of intravenous therapy, we have realized continuous improvement in compliance with intravenous therapy policies and procedures. Problems with equipment and the use of equipment have been identified, leading to changes in equipment and procedures.

Increased Awareness and Appreciation for QA

Through the education efforts and demonstrated improvement in patient care, there is increased awareness about QA at the unit staff level. QA is no longer thought of as something that is done by someone else in an office, nor does it have the "police" image it used to have. Most staff members are able to verbalize the QA activities that are occurring on their units and can recognize the different steps in the monitoring and evaluation process.

Participation in QA activities has been included in performance standards as well. As emphasized, the PQA directs the power of the individual nurse to positively influence patient care outcomes. The simultaneous embodiment of that power and influence in defining clinical practice is evident in unit and/or specialty care job descriptions. At the CCF, the framework for each position was set at the Division level through the delineation of four to seven key performance responsibilities and related criteria for each job category. However, the definition of clinical practice standards via individualization of the criteria on any given unit or specialty was written by the clinical experts of the unit. Some head nurses chose to involve all personnel, if they had a staff of seasoned practitioners. On other units, where there were fewer experienced personnel, head nurses assembled a smaller group of beginning practitioners to work with preceptors and clinical instructors. The result of this activity yielded specific clinical performance expectations that differed according to the nursing care requirements of each specialty population. Most important, the staff set the direction for those performance criteria.

CONCLUSION

In a dynamic health care environment, it is prudent for models for ongoing evaluation to remain in concert with the internal environment and the external initiatives that are setting the direction for measuring the quality and appropriateness of care. As an open-system model responsive to the environment of the organization and the health care community, the PQA is both congruent with the 10-step process for M & E mandated by the Joint Commission and supportive of continuous improvement. The development, implementation, and utilization of this model have been instrumental in helping all nursing staff at the CCF assume responsibility for and contribute to quality patient outcomes.

REFERENCES

Charns, M.P., & Schaefer, M.J. (1983). *Healthcare organizations, a model for management.* Engelwood Cliffs, NJ: Prentice-Hall.

Deming, W.E. (1982). *Quality, productivity, and competitive position.* Boston: MIT Center for Advanced Engineering Study.

Joint Commission on Accreditation of Healthcare Organizations. (1986). *Monitoring and evaluation in nursing services.* Chicago: Author.

Juran, J.M. (1989). *Juran on leadership for quality.* New York: Free Press.

Nadzam, D.M., & Atkins, P.M. (1987). The pyramid for quality assurance. *Journal of Nursing Quality Assurance, 2,* 13–20.

Walton, M. (1986). *The Deming management model.* New York: Putnam.

8

Using Automated Systems for Quality Assurance

Jean A. Walters, MS, RN, Assistant Vice President, Specialty Care Nursing, *Froedtert Memorial Lutheran Hospital, Milwaukee, Wisconsin*

Computerization is an established fact of life in the United States today, and its use is becoming more and more prevalent in health care institutions. Quality assurance (QA) and computerization are naturals for nurses. Our founder, Florence Nightingale, made extensive use of statistics and graphed her information (manually, of course) to evaluate the nursing care given in the Crimea. Therefore, given our past and our present, it seems natural that computers and QA should go hand in hand. Despite the seemingly natural fit of computers with QA, research indicates that registered nurses tend to be somewhat undecided in their attitudes toward their use of computers (McConnell, Summers O'Shea, & Kirchhoff, 1989, p. 39). This research, however, dealt primarily with staff nurses and not specifically with QA professionals who, in the opinion of this author, use computers frequently for QA activities. The attitude of staff nurses is important nonetheless for QA coordinators to consider in their efforts to involve staff in QA activities, some of which may be computerized.

DECISION TO USE COMPUTERIZATION FOR QA ACTIVITIES

But even with history and this natural fit, nursing managers, QA coordinators, and staff nurses (all individuals henceforth referred to as QA professionals in this chapter) must answer several more questions in deciding whether to use comput-

Special thanks to Carol Norris, Patient Care Systems Coordinator at Froedtert Memorial Lutheran Hospital, for her assistance and direction both in writing this chapter and in the use of computerized quality assurance applications on a day-to-day basis, and to Carol Porth, RN, PhD, Research Consultant, Froedtert Memorial Lutheran Hospital, and Associate Professor, University of Wisconsin-Milwaukee, School of Nursing, for her assistance in computerizing and analyzing the medication error survey. Extra special thanks to my family: my husband, Bob, and my children, Tanya and Tate, for their ongoing love and support in this and all my projects.

erization for QA efforts. These are the steps that will help the QA professional make that decision:

1. Define in writing exactly what will be measured, studied, or monitored.
2. Decide if the health care institution's philosophy supports computerization.
3. Decide if time will be saved by use of computerization.
4. Decide if money will be saved by use of computerization.

Defining in writing exactly what is the purpose of the study will provide the basics for determining whether it can be computerized. From these basics, the answer to the next three areas can help decide if computerization should be planned. The institution's philosophy on computer usage is very important. Evaluate the number of computers that are available in the institution. See how many other administrators, finance officers, and other department managers accumulate data via computers and use computerized data for executive presentations. Does the health care institution have an institutional information system that can help support a computer application? If frequent computer usage exists in the institution, the philosophy is positive toward increased use of computerization for other projects.

Next, decide if the computer will save time with QA activities. The computer saves time if the activities that will be computerized are frequent and complex and require mathematical calculations and extensive data manipulation. Time saving from computerization is not automatic, however, and the QA user needs to be aware that it takes time to plan a program, have the program written, enter data, generate reports, and maintain the system. Many of these time-consuming tasks may currently be transparent to the QA user who is the recipient of computerized reports.

The next decision is the cost that is involved. Although computer hardware, software, supplies, and entry time cost money, it is important for the QA professional to consider that time is saved by not having to consolidate and format the data manually in different formats. In addition, it is important to remember that there is a vastly expanded capability for analysis when computerization is used over manual systems. This enhanced analytical capability can give the QA professional an expanded ability to measure quality, which is a definite advantage not to be overlooked. Many health care institutions require a cost-benefit study to be conducted prior to purchase of a computer for a new application. This is only reasonable in today's cost-conscious environment and is a good way for the QA professional to validate that the planned project needs to be computerized.

All of these factors need to be considered when the decision is made to computerize a QA application. It is important also for the novice user of computers to begin with a small project. Use of a small project can give the QA professional much experience in learning the capabilities of the computer, information that will be most helpful in future larger applications.

ADVANTAGES OF COMPUTERIZATION

While there are many advantages to computerization for QA, only the main ones will be discussed in this chapter. The fact that we are a computer literate society is a big advantage, as people are interested in and aware of the use of computerized data. QA activities frequently generate a mammoth amount of data, which the computer can easily handle. In addition, the computer can analyze complex relationships. For instance, if the nursing division is interested in evaluating whether medication errors increase when graduate nurses who are not yet registered nurses begin employment in the institution, the QA professional might investigate the following questions:

1. Were more medication errors made by graduate nurses or by registered nurses during a particular time period? The ratio of graduate nurses to registered nurses in the institution could be compared by the computer in analyzing numbers of errors.
2. Were the medication errors made by the graduate nurses more serious than those made by registered nurses?

The severity of errors could be determined by categorizing medication errors into three categories:

1. no impact on patient (i.e., a vitamin given late)
2. moderate impact on patient (i.e., a patient received too much insulin, but patient's blood sugar did not significantly change due to the increased insulin)
3. severe impact on patient (i.e., an overdose of a narcotic, with patient needing a narcotic antagonist to recover)

Correlating these complex relationships would be practically impossible to perform manually, but with the statistical calculations made possible by computerization, they are easily analyzed.

Another advantage of computerization is speedier processing of information, which can result in more timely reporting. The computer can also weight the importance of criteria; for instance, if a QA professional wanted to identify certain criteria that should be met 100% of the time while other criteria should be met only 95% of the time, a simple statistical calculation can weigh the more important criteria more heavily than the less important criteria. Subscores can also be easily calculated by a computer, for better data analysis. For instance, if the nursing division were monitoring several nursing care standards in 1 month, the scores for each standard, such as admission and patient safety standards, could be calculated individually, while calculating in addition a score for the overall compliance. This helps to identify areas where standards are being met very well and other areas where improvement could be made. In the same manner, scores could be tabulated on a nursing-wide basis as well as on a unit-specific basis. This allows each unit to evaluate its score compared with the nursing-wide score. In addition, if QA data are computerized, they can easily be linked with other patient data, such as length of stay, acuity, and diagnosis-related group (DRG) case-mix information. For example, the QA professional might monitor the average acuity of all patients who fell over a 6-month period of time to see if any trends occurred. Perhaps patients with higher acuities might be identified as more apt to fall. In this way, patients at risk could be more easily identified and preventive interventions taken with this group. The QA professional could then monitor, by computerized reports, if these preventive strategies help to reduce falls in the high-risk groups.

DISADVANTAGES OF COMPUTERIZATION

Despite the numerous advantages of computerization, some disadvantages do exist. In the past the charge of dehumanization of patient care studies with computer use has been levied. It is important to build in ways to prevent dehumanization, for several reasons—first, to maintain the tie with the actual patient or case data and, second, to be able to track any serious issue that needs follow-up. For instance, if patient identification was not gathered in a study of medication errors, it would be difficult to check back in every instance of errors that resulted in severe patient adverse reactions to determine what caused the error and if appropriate corrective actions were carried out. Information should also be gathered on the caregiver so that the data are available for nurse evaluation. It is important to remember, however, that a significant amount of information needs to be gathered on the care provided by any one nurse in order for the computerized data to be statistically significant. A limited sample will not give an accurate picture of the nurse's overall performance.

Another disadvantage to computerizing QA data has to do with confidentiality. Although confidentiality issues exist when data are tabulated and stored in hard copy, the recent rush of break-ins into computer systems has forced a higher priority to be put on protecting data. This will be discussed in more detail later in this chapter.

A third disadvantage of computerization is that some information cannot be accumulated by the computer in a form that lends itself well to analysis. Qualitative data, such as comments, cannot be captured for entry on a computer in a numerical format, which requires a "no" or "nonapplicable" answer format or another format that's easily analyzed.

Data entry and system maintenance must also be considered when using computers; QA professionals may not have staff for these purposes. Such a lack of staff can be resolved in different ways. Of course, additional staff can be requested in the budgetary process. Frequently, however, the QA professional will need to be more resourceful and may look to other departments, such as the institutional information systems, as well as other areas, like the volunteer department, for assistance. We have successfully trained a number of volunteers to do simple data entry and system maintenance tasks for our computer-based QA programs. However, it is important to keep in mind that the confidentiality of the patient must be respected at all times when using other staff for data entry. This can be accomplished by using medical record numbers and employee code numbers only.

A final disadvantage to use of computers for QA purposes is that many QA professionals may not be computer/computer programming literate and may need to increase their knowledge of these systems through study and experience using them, to use them effectively. The institutional information system can be a resource for learning and for applications.

HARDWARE AND SOFTWARE DECISIONS

After the decision has been made to use computerization with QA data, the decision on what hardware and software to buy comes next. The first decision should really be the choice of software to use with the desired application. However, frequently the QA professional does not have the luxury of choosing the software first. For instance, the health care institution may have standardized hardware and software for use by its departments, either purchased on its own or received as a gift as a complement to a major business contract, and so the choice may be out of the QA professional's hands; users must adapt to this decision in order to receive ongoing computer support. This is an important consideration for the QA professional, since a back-up system will be needed in order to save data, and since the QA professional will occasionally (or more frequently!) need help to debug program glitches, times when the program doesn't work.

If the decision on hardware and software has not been made, the QA professional should choose software first. However, since hardware choices often have already been made by the institution, hardware considerations will be discussed first.

The most comprehensive computer system is a mainframe, an interdepartmentally integrated computer system with multiple users, high-volume data entry ability, and applications created for high-level institutional use (Christensen & Stearns, 1984, pp. 7–8). A mainframe is a very expensive and extensive computer system, and it may not be available for the QA professional's use as programming changes may be costly and time consuming. The mainframe system tends to be less flexible; a program change needs to be planned months to weeks in advance and may also encompass a fee for the change. The mainframe, however, does permit one access to other patient-related data, such as admitting, discharge, transfer, length of stay, patient classification, and other data, making them easier to correlate with QA data. Data from the mainframe can also be downloaded to either a mini- or a microcomputer for greater flexibility.

A frequently used type of hardware for QA is the microcomputer or personal computer (PC). The PC may be used in several different formats: It may stand alone, meaning it is not integrated with another computer, or it may be tied in with other computers so that data can be shared from one computer to another (i.e., it may be part of a network).

Frequently, however, PCs are not directly tied in with stored patient-related and financial information, which is usually on a mainframe computer, making it difficult to integrate QA data with patient data unless patient data are downloaded from the mainframe and entered into the PC. Advantages of PCs are that they are less expensive and more flexible than a mainframe. Changes are made with relative ease, compared with making changes on a mainframe.

A minicomputer is another excellent option for use with QA data. A minicomputer combines the advantages of a PC with the advantages of a mainframe system. Minicomputers perform all the functions of a mainframe but at a lower cost, while allowing multiple users.

Whichever hardware is used, it is important to remember that the system should optimally provide the following:

1. a hard disk for long-term storage of QA data
2. tape storage, permitting data to be looked at when needed
3. enough storage capacity to maintain 5 years' worth of data online (This allows the QA specialist to look at trends over a period of time, for year-to-date, or for month-to-date, compared with prior years.)
4. ability to accommodate multiple concurrent users (Any large application should offer this capability.)
5. remote terminals sited away from the QA office, preferably at the location of data gathering, to allow the person gathering the data to immediately enter it (These remote terminals need to be limited in number, and access to them should be controlled. Security should be provided at both a terminal level and a user level.)

Planning for the software, as previously indicated, ideally comes before planning for the hardware. One of the most important factors in deciding on the software is the flexibility of the software program to meet the needs of the QA activities. In addition, the QA professional must decide to either purchase a software package or create one. There are advantages and disadvantages to both decisions.

Purchasing a Prepackaged Software Program

There are a number of advantages to purchasing a prepackaged software program, especially in terms of saving time. For one thing, working with a programmer to design a QA application program is time consuming, so purchasing a prepackaged one saves time.

Another advantage is that the validity and reliability of the tool probably have already been determined for the user, which is an important consideration for QA applications. The purchaser should investigate a program's validity and reliability prior to purchasing it, to be assured of having an accurate tool. Another distinct advantage of purchasing a tool already in use is that frequently, especially if it involves a large application and has experienced wide sales, it may permit the QA professional to have access to regional and/or national data statistics for comparative purposes. It is, of course, important to compare your data with your own past experience, but it adds a depth of comparison when the QA professional is able to compare the institution's results with other institutions' statistics. For instance, the medication error rate is one statistic for which it is very useful to have comparative statistics. The medication error rate in any institution can always be improved, but it is difficult to set a threshold when only looking at the institution's past rate. Therefore, having access to regional and/or national statistics, especially those that deal with reasons for errors, types of medications involved, and other data, is very important.

There are disadvantages, however, to purchasing a preprogrammed QA application. Many times cost is high, as the purchaser is paying for the programming and its tested reliability and validity, training and installation, and many other services. Some quality monitoring applications not only have an initial fee but an ongoing monthly or yearly leasing fee, an upgrade fee, and a maintenance fee. Therefore, the QA professional needs to recommend and purchase the appropriate application with an eye toward using the institution's funds efficiently. In addition, the QA professional needs to plan his or her budgetary proposals in advance, in order to have enough funds to make such a substantial financial investment.

Another disadvantage of purchasing a prepackaged QA program is that the program frequently cannot be modified for institutional needs. This can be a distinct disadvantage, as it is inevitable that the QA professional will need or want to modify and enhance the program to meet institutional needs, something not possible for certain prepackaged QA programs.

HOW TO CHOOSE A QA SOFTWARE PACKAGE

As the purchase of preprogrammed software can be very costly and engender other disadvantages, it is important for the QA professional to have predetermined criteria with which to choose a software package. Stevens (1988, pp. 458–460) has identified some of these criteria, which will now be described.

Learn As Much As Possible about All Your Options

Assessing all the different options available is very important for the QA professional to make an informed decision. One way to find out about many different software programs is to attend a QA conference and view the vendors' exhibit area. This is a way to see many vendors at one time and to identify those of interest. QA professionals can, by having clearly identified the purpose of the software, scan and identify those software packages that are applicable for the desired purpose. Vendors are frequently very willing to bring their products to the health care institution for the QA professional and a committee to assess. Another way to define different software options is to contact other QA professionals. QA networking groups are very helpful in discussing different software applications. A third way to get ideas about options is to read magazines and periodicals that deal with QA; one may examine the advertisements of QA software vendors or articles on different applications and contact their authors.

Define a List of Criteria with Which To Compare the Products

The following list is very helpful and a starting point for the QA professional's own specific list of criteria.

Ease of Use Initially and for New Users

It's important for the QA professional to carefully assess the ease with which the software application can be used. Frequently sales representatives, who are very familiar with their application, give an inordinately simple demonstration of the ease with which the program can be used. The QA professional should ask to use the application during the demonstration to ''get a feel for'' the ease with which the application can be used. It is especially important to review ease of use for new, inexperienced computer users. If a QA professional is a new user, it's important for him or her to have a comfortable feeling of ease in use of the product, or to have a resource person on staff who can quickly acquire that ease and assist the QA professional in use of the application.

Ease of Use for Experienced Infrequent Users

This criterion is slightly different from the first criterion in that there are some QA applications that call for use on a 3-, 6-, or 12-month basis. Over an extended period of time, one may forget how to work some of these applications. Therefore, the number of help screens and documentation resources that are available is very important. This directly leads us into the next criterion.

Documentation References

A sign of a high-quality QA application is a well-developed, easy-to-follow documentation reference manual. This manual will be used frequently by the new user in the beginning and will be an ongoing source of support for the QA professional and other new users. The QA professional should examine the documentation resources to follow one example through to its conclusion. If this can be easily done, the system is well designed. A large number of on-screen helps is also another sign of quality in a QA software package. Frequently these helps explain codes or give direction to the user when the user is unable to proceed further.

Flexibility in Data That Can Be Collected

The QA professional should be able to gather multiple types of data with the software package and, more important, be able to individualize these data to the institution's specific uses. This ability to adapt the software to the institution's needs is sometimes not available, but when it is, it is a definite asset to the QA professional and one criterion that should strongly recommend a program for purchase.

Time Needed for Data Input

The time needed for data input is important to consider as sometimes, especially with new applications, this time might be needed from the QA professional himself or herself, the secretarial support for the professional, staff nurses, and sometimes untrained volunteer staff. Therefore, the data input time is costly and must be considered in the overall applicability of the package. It's also important to determine if data entry time increases as more data are accumulated in the system. This has occurred with several applications in the writer's institution and can considerably increase the amount of time and resources needed for data entry.

Time Taken To Produce the Analyses and Reports

The QA professional must review the reports generated to note their detail and the ease with which an analysis can be accomplished. It is important for reports to be kept as simple as possible for user friendliness and ease in analyzing and interpreting results. Therefore, lengthy reports are not necessarily the best type. In addition, the QA professional must question the vendor to determine the length of time it takes to produce reports; on occasion, reports, even if they do not appear to be lengthy, take a substantial amount of time to process and produce, and the computer cannot be used during the time when reports are being created. If that is the case, the QA professional should investigate the ease with which the computer can be programmed to print reports overnight. Even if at present the QA professional does not see a problem with having reports that take hours to print, if in the future the QA professional expects to use more applications, this will become a problem.

Security and Confidentiality

Any time QA data are compiled, security is a factor to consider. This is particularly an issue in today's computer literate society. The national press has been discussing the ease with which computer network break-ins occur. Precautions must be put in place to prevent such security breakdowns. The QA professional should question the vendor regarding the number of different levels of security that are built into a QA software package. Staff who will only be inputting data will need the most basic security level. Staff who will be analyzing and working with the data will need a higher security level, and, finally, staff who will be problem solving program quirks will need the highest level. It is desirable to have at minimum three levels of security built into the computer program. Confidentiality is also an important issue, which has been discussed previously in this chapter.

Training and Support

The amount of training and support that comes with purchase of the QA computer software is important to assess. Whenever a software package is purchased, it should be used to its ultimate, and this cannot occur without effective training. The QA professional should determine the maximum number of staff who can be trained as part of the QA software purchase and should identify those staff who will be most helpful in ongoing support and use of the software. The QA professional should also, in checking references of other users of the QA package, ask if the training period allocated by the vendor was sufficient for those users. If not, the QA professional should negotiate to increase the amount of training time to ensure staff competence in using the system. The amount of ongoing support is also crucial for the QA professional to determine, because every computerized system has breakdowns, some minor and some major. The QA professional should determine the amount of in-house support for both the hardware and the software in evaluating the amount of vendor support that is necessary. If ongoing vendor support is not included as part of the purchase and there is no in-house support available, the QA professional should negotiate some ongoing vendor support as part of the purchase agreement. Either way, it is crucial that the QA professional determine, prior to purchase of the software package, where ongoing support will be obtained.

Dependability and Experience of Supplier

The dependability and experience of the supplier are important issues for the QA professional to determine. As a rule of thumb, the more well known the vendor, the more reliable the package should be. This is not to say, however, that a new vendor should be overlooked if the software package seems to meet the specifications desired. The QA professional should ask for and check at least two references. Checking several references should give the QA professional a good idea of the reliability of the product. The QA professional need not check references unless he or she is seriously considering purchase of the software package. One reason for checking references is to determine how other institutions have utilized the software package. Frequently, in use of a program, the QA professional learns how to more fully adapt the program outside of its intended use. The QA professional should specifically ask about enhanced usage when making reference calls. If the software package is relatively new and there are few, if any, existing applications, the QA professional should then check on the experience and reliability of the supplier as one criterion with which to compare the applicability of the software program. A vendor's reputation frequently speaks for itself and will give excellent information about the quality of any new application.

Once the QA professional has identified several programs and made reference calls, the professional should seriously consider making site visits at one or two user sites. Site visits will provide an opportunity to see the program in action as well as to determine how the program is being used. In determining who should accompany the QA professional for site visits, one or more of these individuals should be strongly considered as candidates:

1. The nursing computer consultant in your institution: This individual can be a valuable resource in determining the ease with which the package can be used.
2. The director of the institution's information systems: This person understands the ins and outs of computerization in a more in-depth manner and can give valuable information on use of the computerized system.
3. The nursing administrator: This person will be a valuable advocate in allocating funds to purchase the program if he or she realizes the full extent of the program application.
4. The finance administrator: Financial staff have used computers for many years and more fully realize the analytical capability and the reporting capabilities of computerized systems.

Overall, the time and money invested in site visits will be well worth the effort when the QA application is used fully and effectively on an ongoing basis.

Modification of Input/Output

The ability of the software program to be modified for individual health care institution use is very important for the QA professional to consider. As previously indicated, once a computer is used for an application, the user frequently identifies adaptations, modifications, and other uses for the computerized program. Therefore, having the ability to modify both the input and the output for the organization's use is very important. Simple touches, such as having the institution's name printed out on reports and other similar touches, will make the software package be much more accepted and utilized at the QA professional's institution.

Data Storage Capacity

The QA professional should assess the amount of data that can be maintained on the system—that is, the number of years data can be kept online. This is very important for gathering information on trends. The ideal system should be able to maintain 5 years of data online (after 5 years, the data may become outdated). The QA professional can use this 5 years' worth of data in several ways: having the previous year-to-date and/or previous year's month-to-date information printed next to current information, for data comparison on a month-to-month basis, or having reports generated periodically throughout the year, such as every 6 months and at year end, that compare with the previous year's data to permit trends to be spotted. For instance, the rate from year to year of medication errors per 1000 patient days is important to monitor, and it would be important to have data from the past several years available for comparative purposes (as rate per 1000 patient days takes into account the change in patient census).

Capability of Interfacing with Other Computer Systems

The capability of interfacing with other computer systems is very important, as statistics necessary for comparison may be stored on another computer. Therefore, you may need to download certain data, such as DRG case-mix data, average length of stay, patient acuity, and other information, onto the computer with the QA application. The QA professional should assess the current computerized system in the institution to identify which would have data that may need to be integrated with the QA application. Then the QA professional should question the vendor concerning whether these specific systems can be interfaced.

Determine a Weighting System for the Criteria

For each of these previously mentioned criteria, the QA professional should determine a weight, for instance, from zero to five, with zero being useless for the purpose and five being excellent. The QA professional can then rate each criterion and add the total weightings to determine the overall applicability of the software package. Once the rating of all the systems has been determined, the next step is to arrange demonstrations of the highest-ranked packages to gather more information. Determining the score for each proposed software package is important to help narrow down the selection for purchase.

CREATING INSTITUTION-SPECIFIC SOFTWARE

While many QA professionals will feel more comfortable purchasing a pre-programmed package, the professional should not rule out creation of an institution-specific QA application. The main advantage of creating your own software package is that it will meet your own needs; it is not often that a packaged QA application meets every need or desire that the QA professional has. A second advantage is that your own application can be changed or modified as necessary in the future. This is an excellent advantage because, as previously stated, with use the QA professional will probably identify needed enhancements. For instance, the writer's institution's standards of care quality monitoring system uses a randomized auditor selection process. Each nurse in the hospital is listed in the computer as a possible auditor. Because this demographic information is available on each nurse, it was felt that the software package could be used to also gather other information about each nurse, such as inservice attendance, outside education attendance, cardiopulmonary resuscitation certification status, preceptor status, and information on type of orientation. This is all useful information for the institution's education department.

There are, however, disadvantages to creating your own program. First, the QA professional needs to have access to computer-programming resources. These resources may be obtained from internal institutional resources, such as the institutional information system or a nurse who has programming skills, or from a computer consultant hired from outside the institution. In any case the financial cost of employing the programmer needs to be considered. Although internal resources may not actually bill for their services, their time constitutes a cost to the institution. However, since the application is to the institution's benefit, there may be a positive cost-benefit ratio in the end. If an internal resource is used, the QA professional can most likely count on more time being required to finish the program. Usually internal computer programmers have a variety of other projects that they are working on at the same time as the QA application, and since they usually report to an administrator different from the one the QA professional reports to, the QA professional may not be able to reshift the priority of their assignments.

If the QA professional wishes to contract with an external computer programmer, he or she will need to have a budget with which to hire this consultant. As a rule of thumb, an institution should dedicate at least 1% of its annual budget to QA resources. Part of this 1% could be used by the QA professional to hire a computer programmer. An external consultant usually will complete a programming assignment in a much more timely fashion than an internal programmer will, as the external consultant is dependent on completing projects for payment. Therefore, using an external consultant may be the answer for the QA professional who wants an application completed by a certain time.

One big disadvantage to creating your own program is that the QA professional does not have access to any regional or national data for comparison purposes. This can be a distinct disadvantage to the QA professional who wants to compare his or her results with other results. Another disadvantage to creating your own program is that it can become a costly venture. The computer programmer, whether internal or external, may have underestimated the time needed to write the application, and therefore a long time may elapse until its completion.

If the QA professional chooses to create his or her own package, the following steps can help: First, learn the type of computer systems available at your institution to determine current information access and integration. Strive to integrate clinical, administrative, and patient information as much as possible in your applications.

Second, specify your goals. The more specific information you can give on goals, the better able the programmer will be to carry out your desired program. For example, do not just say that you wish to "measure incident reports." A much more specific statement would be "compare incident report data broken down by all types (medication errors, falls, procedures/equipment problems, etc.) for each month with the number of patient days; compare the month averages with the year-to-date averages and give a semiannual and annual average." In specifying your goals, determine which type of data you will be monitoring, where the data come from, and the ease with which the data can be obtained. Define your analysis in writing to make sure it is comprehensible and understandable. Work with your programmers to clearly define your goals and the desired analysis.

Third, determine who will enter data into the computerized program and what the source document will be for data entry. The source document will need to be more specific if less-trained staff, such as volunteers, will be used for data entry. Be sure that the source document is simple and easy to interpret.

Fourth, plan your reports. Remember to keep them simple and easy to understand. Minimize the number of reports to only those that will be usable either to the internal QA staff or to their audience (nursing division, board of directors, etc.). Plan the scoring for your reports, and keep it as simple as possible. You do want to be able to do all of the complex analytical statistics desired, but plan to use the simplest statistical device that will give information desired.

Fifth, work with your consultant to build validity and reliability into your tool. Make sure that your tool is based on standards, that your study is comprehensive, and that you have a specific standard of measurement built into the tool. The tool must relate to what it is measuring, be objective, identify problems, and provide timely information. Each question must be clear and definitive. Consider how inter-rater reliability can be built into ongoing usage of the tool. Many of these validity and reliability standards can be tested during a pilot of the tool.

Sixth, in working with the programmer, one simple rule applies: Remember the ultimate value of the software application to the user. Keep every aspect of the applicable as simple as possible, from the data entry tool to the screens to the reports.

EXAMPLES OF COMPUTERIZED QA APPLICATIONS

Computerized QA applications can exist in any type of health care institution, from hospitals to ambulatory care to long-term care or home care. In whatever setting these applications exist, it is important for QA professionals to work with professionals in other related areas as much as possible. For instance, the QA department may work with utilization management, risk management, and infection control staff in conducting studies, or at the very least in determining mutual data elements that all these areas may be studying. By having these related disciplines give input into the design of computerized QA applications, the institution reduces duplication, increases productivity, and has increased information available for sharing among related disciplines.

In a hospital, a number of different applications might exist. The QA professional may computerize a system of universal indicators, monitored on an ongoing basis by a variety of departments. Such indicators might include patient falls that resulted in injury, patient falls that did not result in injury, medication errors that resulted in injuries, number of incident reports, and the like. The threshold for the hospital can be programmed into the software, and any outliers that exceed the threshold can be identified with an asterisk by the computer. In addition, each department can get a reading of its monthly results as compared to the hospital-wide results. This gives each department a perspective on how the quality of care in its department compares with that of other hospital departments.

Table 8-1 shows the computerized report of certain indicators for a pulmonary cardiology department of a hospital. The patient satisfaction questionnaire results were not available in the first quarter of 1989, as the survey tool was being revised. There were no complaints in January and February, so the threshold of zero for both complaint categories was not exceeded. Sick hours/month and budgeted worked hours are compared in the last statistics to determine if sufficient staff were available to provide consistent care. The standard is 0.05% or less, and this was not exceeded in either month. This department's sick hours constituted 1.34% of the total hospital sick hours. This percent of hospital total number can be evaluated monthly to see if any increases occurred, but the department percent must also take into account the number of staff in that department. Although only four indicators

Table 8-1 Hospital-Wide QA Report

Pulmonary Cardiology Rt	Threshold	Jan	Feb	Mar	Apr	May	Jun
Pt Satis Quest Results	80.00%	n/a	n/a				
# Pt/Family Complaints	0	0	0				
# MD/Other Dept Complaints	0	0	0				
Sick Hours/Mo		50	61				
No. Budgeted Worked Hours		3953.73	3953.73	3953.73	3953.73	3953.73	3953.73
% Sick Hours to Budgeted	0.05%	0.01%	0.01%	0.00%	0.00%	0.00%	0.00%

Source: Courtesy of Froedtert Memorial Lutheran Hospital, Milwaukee, WI.

are monitored in this example, one distinct advantage is that the same data are gathered for all hospital departments, which makes comparing one department to all others possible.

The QA professional may also computerize incident report data (Table 8-2). This example provides data for 1 month only, as the system was planned to be initiated in July, 1989. Over time, information on the report will give valuable trending information to the QA professional. The computerized program also automatically tabulates the statistics on the report, a task that previously took much of the QA professional's time.

Computerizing incident report data would allow the QA professional to obtain specific information on different types of incidents, such as patient falls. The QA professional may wish to investigate the times of day falls occurred, what the patient was doing at the time of the fall, what units the falls occurred on, whether the patient had been restrained, whether siderails had been up, and other similar information. The ability to investigate different aspects of an incident helps in identifying problems for follow-up investigations.

Another example of computerized incident report data facilitating QA investigations may be produced by a nursing manager who wishes to compare the unit length of stay with the nosocomial infection rate to see if patients who have a longer length of stay (beyond the average for that unit) have a higher nosocomial infection rate than patients with an average length of stay. This information would help the nursing manager and unit staff plan appropriate interventions if problems were identified.

Hexum and Bachman (1987, p. 72–76) wrote about a decentralized QA study conducted by staff nurses on a unit using a portable computer or data entry at the site of data accumulation. The computer was lightweight, the size of a brief case with a flip-up screen. It was battery powered and rechargeable, and staff nurses carried it to the bedside to gather and enter data immediately, and returned it to the nursing manager for data tabulation and analysis. This innovative use of the computer streamlined data entry, eliminated the need for a data entry form, and oriented the nursing staff to the benefits of using computers for QA activities.

Jul	Aug	Sep	Oct	Nov	Dec	YTD	Avg	% Total
						0	0	
						0	0	0.00%
						0	0	0.00%
						111.00	55.50	1.34%
3953.73	3953.73	3953.73	3953.73	3953.73	3953.73	47444.8	3953.73	2.89%
0.00%	0.00%	0.00%	0.00%	0.00%	0.00%	0.02%	.00%	

The power of the computer to manipulate data can also be used for correlating and comparing information, as was done by the author in an analysis of medication errors. Recently, the nursing care evaluation committee at Froedtert Memorial wanted to study medication errors, in an effort to reduce them. The first step was to gather information on the actual practice of reporting medication errors. The committee wondered whether nurses were under-reporting medication errors as defined by policy and procedure. The committee designed and conducted a medication error survey (see Exhibit 8-1) during a medication awareness inservice. Sixty-four percent of the possible respondents (n = 284) completed the survey, and the results were tabulated with use of the computer, the programs having been written by an in-house computer consultant and a nursing researcher with whom the hospital contracted for services.

One point became evident early in working with the nurse researcher to analyze the medication error survey results: It would have been very helpful to have had the nurse researcher review the survey tool prior to its use (we brought the nurse researcher into the process after the survey had been conducted). For example, had the nurse respondent listed continuous data, such as length of time as a nurse or length of employment at our hospital, instead of fixed-range options, the data could have been manipulated more extensively. It also would have been helpful to have piloted the tool with 10 or more individuals prior to usage. That way, changes could have been made to improve the tool. For instance, it would have been better to rate the major perceived causes of medication errors on a scale rather than merely identify them as a major perceived cause. A rating system would have given a more sophisticated way of identifying the major perceived causes of medication errors that exist at Froedtert.

When the computer run of the statistical data was reviewed with the nurse researcher, it was determined that many data were missing. For instance, nurses in some areas, such as surgery, do not give medications. Their responses, however, were tallied along with those of nurses who do give medications. While indeed they may have good perceptions of what causes medication errors, their lack of knowledge and use of the current medication system made their perceptions less

Table 8-2 QA Report of Incident Report Data

Incident Description	Month Total	% of Total Incidents	Rate/1000 Pt Days	Jan	Feb	Mar	Apr
Fall	34	29.57	5.99	0	0	0	0
Other accident or injury	2	1.74	0.35	0	0	0	0
Total falls & other injuries	36	31.30	6.34	0	0	0	0
Scheduling not drawn	1	0.87	0.18	0	0	0	0
Delayed results	1	0.87	0.18	0	0	0	0
Mislabeled specimen—nursing	0	0.00	0.00	0	0	0	0
Other lab errors	7	6.09	1.23	0	0	0	0
Lab errors	9	7.83	1.59	0	0	0	0
NSG interdepartment comm. breakdown	1	0.87	0.18	0	0	0	0
MD interdept. comm. breakdown	0	0.00	0.00	0	0	0	0
NSG/MD interdept. comm. breakdown	0	0.00	0.00	0	0	0	0
CSC interdept. breakdown	4	3.48	0.70	0	0	0	0
Other interdept. comm. breakdown	4	3.48	0.70	0	0	0	0
Interdepartment communication breakdown	9	7.83	1.59	0	0	0	0
Incorrect narcotic count	1	0.87	0.18	0	0	0	0
Incorrect OR count	6	5.22	1.06	0	0	0	0
Incorrect narcotics/OR count	7	6.09	1.23	0	0	0	0
Treatment problem	1	0.87	0.18	0	0	0	0
Procedure problem	9	7.83	1.59	0	0	0	0
Equipment-related problem	5	4.35	0.88	0	0	0	0
Other treatment/procedure problem	0	0.00	0.00	0	0	0	0
Treatment/procedure problem	15	13.04	2.64	0	0	0	0
Patient/personnel security problem	1	0.87	0.18	0	0	0	0
Valuables missing	6	5.22	1.06	0	0	0	0
Miscellaneous	9	7.83	1.59	0	0	0	0
TOTAL OF ALL TYPES	92	80	16.21	0	0	0	0

Note: CSC = clinical system communicator (unit clerk); OR = operating room.

Source: Courtesy of Froedtert Memorial Lutheran Hospital, Milwaukee, WI.

accurate than those of nurses who actually gave medications. Therefore, the survey results were reviewed to determine which surveys should be eliminated from the analysis. This task was quickly accomplished because the data were on a computer.

In data analysis, the computer was helpful initially in determining the frequency with which each of the questions was answered. This task alone would have taken a long time if performed manually. Each survey was given a number, and a volunteer entered the data into the computer. Having the data on the computer allowed some initial observations to be made. For instance, the options in question 7 were all legitimate instances when, according to our hospital's policies and

May	Jun	Jul	Aug	Sep	Oct	Nov	Dec	Average Month	YTD Total	Last Year YTD
0	0	34	0	0	0	0	0	4.86	34	0
0	0	2	0	0	0	0	0	0.29	2	0
0	0	36	0	0	0	0	0	5.14	36	0
0	0	1	0	0	0	0	0	0.14	1	0
0	0	1	0	0	0	0	0	0.14	1	0
0	0	0	0	0	0	0	0	0.00	0	0
0	0	7	0	0	0	0	0	1.00	7	0
0	0	9	0	0	0	0	0	1.29	9	0
0	0	1	0	0	0	0	0	0.14	1	0
0	0	0	0	0	0	0	0	0.00	0	0
0	0	0	0	0	0	0	0	0.00	0	0
0	0	4	0	0	0	0	0	0.57	4	0
0	0	4	0	0	0	0	0	0.57	4	0
0	0	9	0	0	0	0	0	1.29	9	0
0	0	1	0	0	0	0	0	0.14	1	0
0	0	6	0	0	0	0	0	0.86	6	0
0	0	7	0	0	0	0	0	1.00	7	0
0	0	1	0	0	0	0	0	0	1	0
0	0	9	0	0	0	0	0	1.29	9	0
0	0	5	0	0	0	0	0	0	5	0
0	0	0	0	0	0	0	0	0	0	0
0	0	15	0	0	0	0	0	2.14	15	0
0	0	1	0	0	0	0	0	0.14	1	0
0	0	6	0	0	0	0	0	0.86	6	0
0	0	9	0	0	0	0	0	1.29	9	0
0	0	92	0	0	0	0	0	13.14	92	0

procedures, a nurse should have completed an incident report for a medication error. However, only 13% of respondents indicated that they would complete an incident report for all of the reasons listed. It was reassuring, however, to note that all the respondents indicated that they would complete a medication incident report when the medication error involved a potentially life-threatening situation for the patient or if the medication was a drug vital to patient treatment.

As indicated by the previous example, analyzing the responses to the survey questions gave a good indication of actual nursing practice. Nursing administration felt that this information was invaluable, and a task force composed of staff nurses, nursing managers, pharmacists, and QA professionals was formed to

Exhibit 8-1 Medication Error Survey

The Nursing Care Evaluation Committee is studying medication errors in an effort to reduce them. Your input in completing this survey will help us in this process.

THERE ARE NO RIGHT OR WRONG ANSWERS. We would like you to answer these questions with the way you are currently practicing—not with the answer you think is correct. YOUR ANSWERS ON THIS SURVEY ARE TOTALLY ANONYMOUS. All responses will be tallied and printed in an upcoming issue of *Primarily Nursing*.

1. How long have you been a nurse?

    a. _____ under one year
    b. _____ over one–five years
    c. _____ over five–ten years
    d. _____ ten plus years

2. How long have you worked as a nurse at Froedtert?

    a. _____ under one year
    b. _____ over one–three years
    c. _____ over three plus years

3. How old are you? (OPTIONAL)

    a. _____ 20–34 years
    b. _____ 35–44 years
    c. _____ 45 + years

4. a. *At the beginning of the week*, do you check all of your patients' MARs at the beginning of your shift to record meds to be given?

                          Yes   No

    b. *In the middle of the week*, do you check all of your patients' MARs at the beginning of your shift to record meds to be given?

                          Yes   No

5. How do you organize your assignment to plan for patient medication administration:

    a. _____ use activity sheet
    b. _____ combine all meds on one work sheet
    c. _____ don't use any sheet
    d. _____ other _____

6. What do you think are the major causes of med errors here at FMLH?

    a. _____ system problems (specify) _____
    _____ _____
    b. _____ nurse forgetfulness or oversight
    c. _____ too frequent interruptions of nurse
    d. _____ unclear MAR
    e. _____ own disorganization
    f. _____ nurse being too busy

continues

Exhibit 8-1 continued

     g. _____ med given over ½ hour late because of arrival time from Pharmacy

     h. _____ others (specify) _____

     _____

7. Check when you would complete an incident report?

     a. _____ any med given more than ½ hour before or ½ hour after scheduled time

     b. _____ a once a day med given more than ½ hour before or ½ hour after scheduled time

     c. _____ a med given one or more hours after discontinuation

     d. _____ a med given by wrong route but with correct dosage

     e. _____ an underdosage of ordered med

     f. _____ a med not given at ordered time because order missed

     g. _____ an omission of drug not vital to patient treatment, such as vitamins, stool-softeners and antacids

     h. _____ an omission of drug vital to patient treatment, such as Digoxin, Lasix, Insulin

     i. _____ meds given over ½ hour late because you were busy with another patient

     j. _____ an incorrect IV solution

     k. _____ an incorrect med administered which doesn't harm the patient

     l. _____ an incorrect med administered to patient which is potentially life-threatening

8. Would you inform the MD when holding the following meds:

     Yes   No

     a. _____ _____ Digoxin when pulse is below 60

     b. _____ _____ Insulin when patient must be NPO for a test

     c. _____ _____ Surfak when patient has diarrhea

     d. _____ _____ Oral cardiac meds when patient is NPO

     e. _____ _____ Oral meds such as antibiotics and hypoglycemic agents when patient NPO for OR

9. How many med errors have you made in the last year? _____

10. How many of your med errors have you reported on incident reports in the last year? _____

11. What do you consider to be a serious med error? _____

_____

_____

_____

12. Other comments on medication administration and/or error rate:

_____

_____

_____

_____

Source: Courtesy of Froedtert Memorial Lutheran Hospital, Milwaukee, WI.

evaluate what changes could be made to reduce medication errors. For example, the most frequently cited reason for not completing an incident report was a once-a-day medication given late (i.e., more than one-half hour before or one-half hour after scheduled time, the hospital's grace period for medication administration). The task force is currently investigating standards at other area hospitals regarding medication administration grace periods and is evaluating whether to extend the hospital's grace period for all medication administration times or for the daily medication administration times only. The preceding example is only one small area that the task force is investigating in order to reduce medication errors, but the computerized data results helped to identify where change might be beneficial and where efforts should be focused.

Some of the answers desired from the medication error survey needed to have statistical analysis other than frequency determination. Several hypotheses were written prior to creation of the medication error survey, to guide our investigation:

Hypothesis 1: Nurses who have worked at Froedtert more than 1 year will have an effective system to organize their assignment and thus prevent medication errors.

Hypothesis 2: Nurses aged 35 years and older will have better clinical routines and therefore will make fewer medication errors.

Hypothesis 3: Nurses who don't check medication administration records (MARs) in the middle of the week make more errors than those who do.

Hypothesis 4: The longer time a nurse, the more likely the nurse will be to report a medication error, whether or not the patient had an adverse reaction.

The task force worked with the nurse researcher to analyze the results of these hypotheses. The hypothesis results were analyzed using the Chi-square statistic with a level of significance of .05 or less.

The data for the first hypothesis were run using the same time frames indicated by question 2 on the Medication Error Survey, i.e. under 1 year, over 1 to 3 years, and over 3 years. The hypothesis was not statistically significant when run using these three time periods; since the time periods did not strictly adhere to the hypothesis, data were re-run by dividing the length of work experience at Froedtert into two categories, under 1 year and over 1 year. The first hypothesis then, was found to be statistically significant. The task force's belief that, at the point of having worked at Froedtert for one year, the nurse should have an effective knowledge of the correct medication administration system which would help prevent errors and which knowledge would not be increased by further work experience, was correct.

Hypothesis 2 was not proven in the first data analysis and was also re-run, again with only two categories—nurses under 35 years old and over 35 years old—rather than three age categories as identified in the Medication Error Survey. Hypothesis 2 was not found to be statistically significant in this re-run. Although nurses 35 years of age and older tended to make less medication errors than those under age 35, the difference was not statistically significant even when the medication error data were analyzed with 0-1 error and 0-2 error categories for the two age ranges.

Hypothesis 3 was not proven. There was no significant difference in the data analysis results between the 100% of nurses who checked the medication administration records at the beginning of the week and those who didn't check them in the middle of the week, in terms of number of medication errors made.

Hypothesis 4 was analyzed by correlating the length of time as a nurse with the number of incident reports indicated on the survey. This correlation was not found to be statistically significant in the first run; however, the results were re-run comparing nurses with less than one year of experience and more than one year of experience as a nurse. With this re-run, hypothesis 4 was statistically significant except the statistics indicated that the longer in nursing, the less likely the nurse would be to report a medication error.

In addition to the ease in re-running these hypotheses, having the data in a computer program allowed us to easily run each variable with every other one and, therefore, led to findings that we had not hypothesized. For instance, it was statistically significant that younger nurses were more apt to use the activity record, our hospital's established mechanism for documenting medication to be administered, than older nurses. We thus hypothesized that older nurses have developed other patterns to document medications to be administered. We also found that older nurses feel that they make more medication errors if they experience frequent interruptions. Therefore, it appears that older nurses may rely on routines and be more apt to make mistakes when these routines are interrupted.

It was also statistically significant that, regardless of age, nurses felt that system problems and nurse forgetfulness were factors in medication errors. It was statistically significant that nurses employed at Froedtert less than 1 year were more likely to report a late medication as an error when it was due to their being too busy.

These statistically significant findings gave the nursing care evaluation committee much information concerning causes of medication errors and indicated directions for improvement. This example of the added significance of computerizing the medication error survey results validates the importance of using a computer to enhance results of similar QA applications.

Numerous other examples exist of computerized QA applications in many areas of nursing. Nursing managers and QA professionals in ambulatory care could correlate the number of return visits with the documentation of appropriate patient education for each specific diagnosis. If a patient continues to need follow-up care when the standard of care suggests that the patient does not need many follow-up visits, a chart review may be necessary to gather more information on why additional visits were needed. The computer, however, can easily tabulate information to help identify outliers that need further follow-up. Computers could also be used by staff nurses in ambulatory care for documentation of care received. The staff could then identify standards of care for different diagnoses and do a focused review from the computerized documentation to see if the standards of care were met. This would help in identifying areas needing improvement and reinforcement.

Staff in home care could use computer programs for generating automatic reminder notices for follow-up checks. For instance, two to three days after a patient has been begun on insulin instruction by the home care nurse, the computer could generate a reminder check indicating that the patient and/or significant other should be able to give the insulin injection by that date. The home care nurse could then indicate the date that the patient and/or significant other was able to give the injection, and a simple computer program could match the patient's outcomes with standards of care to identify any areas needing improvement.

Long-term care nursing managers and QA professionals could computerize medication error information and identify guidelines for threshold comparison. In order to analyze the correlation of each factor with falls, long-term care nurses could monitor the frequency of patient falls on each unit as well as the care class of patients who fell; the shift the patient fell on; the census, number, and type of staff on the unit when the patient fell; and the medications that the patient was receiving at time of fall. For example, if high-acuity patients were the ones who always fell, appropriate preventive nursing interventions could be implemented with all high-acuity patients to reduce risk of falling.

THE FUTURE

The future of computerization for QA efforts will bring a greatly increased usage of computers. The use of terminals at "point of data gathering" will be much more frequent. This means that either portable computer terminals will be used to enter data immediately when they are gathered or that stationary computers will exist at the patient's bedside and that these computers would be available for QA purposes in addition to gathering other patient data, such as vital signs, test treatment results, medications administered, and so forth. Having QA data and other patient data on the same computer will increase the amount of data that are available for QA purposes. It will also increase the ability of QA data to be gathered at the same time that other patient data are gathered and entered into the computer. This will reduce the use of nursing time for only QA activities.

In the future multiple departments will begin to work together much more closely in planning QA studies and data to be gathered. Infection control, QA, risk management, and utilization management will plan computerized systems that meet all areas' needs, in order to reduce duplication and increase efficiency and effectiveness in the institution. Staff in all institutional departments will become more and more aware of QA and will begin to routinely gather QA data on the computer along with their other computerized activities. This increased interest of staff in quality improvement will promote QA activities and will reduce the work needed by nursing managers and QA professionals for QA activities.

Nurses are challenged to learn more about using computers for QA efforts. The use of computers will dramatically increase in the future, and QA professionals must be ready to meet this need.

REFERENCES

Christensen, W.W., & Stearns, E.I. (1984). *Microcomputers in health care management.* Gaithersburg, MD: Aspen Publishers.

Hexum, J., & Bachman, C. (1987). Innovations and excellence. *Journal of Nursing Quality Assurance, 1*(4), 72–76.

McConnell, E.A., Summers O'Shea, S., & Kirchhoff, K.T. (1989). RN attitudes toward computers. *Nursing Management, 20,* 36–40.

Stevens, G. (1988). Selecting computer software packages—a self help guide: Discussion paper. *Journal of the Royal Society of Medicine, 81,* 458–460.

9

Ethical Dilemmas in Nursing Quality Assurance

Mary A. Erickson Megel, PhD, RN, Associate Professor, Parent Child Nursing, College of Nursing, University of Nebraska Medical Center, Omaha, Nebraska

Mary E. Barna Elrod, BSN, RN, Coordinator, Nursing Quality Assurance, University Hospital, University of Nebraska Medical Center, Omaha, Nebraska

An issue that has received little attention in the quality assurance (QA) literature to date is ethics. Perhaps this is related to the relative youth of QA as an area of professional nursing practice. In the 15 years since efforts began to monitor the quality of health care, QA professionals have been preoccupied with such pressing concerns as the development of sound methods, the organization of QA efforts, and the establishment of formal and informal networks for communication and support. Just as nursing continues to develop the professional characteristics of competence, social value, and autonomy, so are nurses involved in the professional development of QA. This development naturally leads to a concern with ethics and the ethical dilemmas inherent in working with nurses and other members of the health team to establish standards and monitor the quality and appropriateness of care provided to clients (Jameton, 1984).

Thus as a function of the ongoing evolution of QA, ethics is an issue whose time has come. This chapter will explore selected ethical dilemmas as they currently occur in QA, discuss resources available for identifying and resolving these dilemmas, and present implications for nursing and other disciplines as they attempt to confront the ethical dilemmas in current QA practice.

ETHICAL DILEMMAS AND PRINCIPLES

Dilemmas

An ethical dilemma exists in a situation that requires making a choice between two (or more) mutually inconsistent courses of action, each of which can be supported by a fundamental ethical principle. In order to act on the basis of one ethical principle, the other courses of action (and their corresponding ethical principles) must be set aside (Beauchamp & Childress, 1979; Jameton, 1984; Purtilo & Cassel, 1981).

What makes the dilemma ethical, as opposed to a legal dilemma or a political dilemma? Three criteria can be used to distinguish ethical courses of action from nonethical action-guides: (1) ethical action-guides are determined by societies to be supreme and over-riding in judgments about actions; (2) ethical action-guides are universal, which requires that all similar cases be treated in the same way; and (3) ethical action-guides have direct reference to the welfare of human beings (Beauchamp & Childress, 1979). No one criterion is sufficient to distinguish ethical from other types of dilemmas; all three criteria must be applied simultaneously.

Determining that ethical dilemmas exist and distinguishing ethical from other types of dilemmas are not easy tasks. For example, the results of QA studies tend to be carefully guarded because of the sensitivity of the information for the health care providers involved. Posting the results of QA studies on bulletin boards in the units of the agency in which the studies were conducted would not create an ethical dilemma in terms of patient confidentiality if the results are displayed in the aggregate; however, this could very well create a political dispute between staff, who may view the results as critical of their performance, and the QA professionals and managers who are attempting to provide feedback to the staff about performance.

Ethics versus Morals

Writers in the area of biomedical ethics often fail to clearly define the terms "ethics" and "morals," and some use the terms interchangeably. Jameton (1984) contrasts these words in terms of professional and personal use, as well as between commitment and inquiry. Professional use of the term "ethics" refers to public, formal statements of rules or values; "morals" refers to a set of values to which an individual is personally committed. In terms of commitment, "morals" refers to values to which one is truly committed; "ethics" refers to a field of systematic inquiry and study. Thus "ethics" tends to be the more formal term, and "morals" more personal.

Maurice and Warrick (1977) present a different approach to distinguishing between morals and ethics. "Ethics," according to the Buddhist philosopher consulted by these authors, reflects an individual's conscious, reasoned, introspective choices, without other emotional motives. Therefore, individuals are responsible for their own ethical decisions. "Morals" refers to duties based upon divine will or other authority; actions based on obedience to rules result.

In order to avoid confusion with personal or religious values, the term "morals" will not be used in this chapter. Instead, "ethics" will be used to refer to the formalized principles based upon reason and rational study that philosophers have defined as having value in our society.

Principles

The principles most often discussed by biomedical ethicists include autonomy, justice, confidentiality, nonmaleficence, beneficence, utility, and fidelity. Each of these principles will be defined, followed by a discussion of ethical dilemmas within QA when two or more of these principles support mutually inconsistent courses of action.

Autonomy refers to self-governance. Individuals are autonomous to the extent that they have relative independence in freely choosing or endorsing specific courses of action based upon their own values, goals, or plans (Benjamin & Curtis, 1981). In health care, the principle of autonomy is honored when patients provide informed consent to invasive procedures or to procedures that involve considerable risk. This means that patients are given all of the information necessary to make a decision, and that the information is communicated in terms that are clearly understood.

Justice is defined in several ways: as desert (people should receive what they deserve); as harmony and balance; as human equality and fairness (Jameton, 1984); and as demonstrated need or the right to a commodity that is necessary to maintain life or dignity (Garrett, Baillie, & Garrett, 1989). Purtilo and Cassel (1981) distinguish three types of justice: (1) distributive, which concerns the comparative treatment of individuals or groups when benefits and burdens are allocated; (2) compensatory, which concerns compensations to individuals or groups who have been wronged; and (3) procedural, which concerns fair treatment of individuals or groups. In health care, the principle of justice is operationalized when patients receive appropriate medical treatment and nursing care for their conditions without regard for their gender, socioeconomic status, age, race, or other characteristics.

Confidentiality refers to truth-telling, the prohibition of telling falsehoods, and the keeping of secrets. Secrets are knowledge that an individual is obligated to conceal and may be of three types: (1) natural secrets, which involve information that would be harmful to an individual if revealed; (2) promised secrets, which is information an individual has promised not to reveal; and (3) professional secrets, which involve information that would harm not only the individual involved but also the profession (Garrett et al., 1989). Within the context of biomedical ethics, the concept of confidentiality typically means that health professionals may not reveal information given to them in confidence unless the client gives permission.

Nonmaleficence means to avoid committing an evil or harmful act (Garrett et al., 1989). In health care, an evil or harmful act usually means an act that could cause pain, suffering, disability, death, or mental damage (Beauchamp & Childress, 1979). In health care, upholding this principle means that health professionals strive to remain current and competent in their practice and review and question the practices of their colleagues to maintain quality of care.

Beneficence means to do good, or to provide benefits to others. In biomedical ethics, beneficence is seen as a duty, not as charity, and involves not only providing appropriate care for patients (the principle of positive beneficence) but also balancing benefits against potential harms (the principle of utility) (Beauchamp & Childress, 1979).

Utility, while related to beneficence, is often discussed as a separate ethical principle, which states that the greatest good or value should be provided to the greatest number of individuals. In this context, the principle of utility is concerned with the results of actions and the attempt to perform acts that will provide the most favorable results for the majority of those involved (Beauchamp & Childress, 1979). Nation-wide immunization programs and mandatory school attendance for American children can be viewed as operationalizations of the principle of utility, since the benefits of such activities are believed to outweigh any potential risk to individuals.

Fidelity refers to faithfulness in relationships between human beings. Some ethicists discuss fidelity in the theological sense of a covenant (Cooper, 1988); others discuss voluntary contract formation between consenting individuals (Beauchamp & Childress, 1979). Purtilo and Cassel (1981) state that a duty of fidelity means keeping promises made to others. Clearly, in health care, promises made to patients about their care by health care providers must be kept in honoring this ethical principle.

Unfortunately, the above descriptions of ethical principles seem overly simplistic in view of the complexity that characterizes today's health care system. The following examples illustrate the types of ethical dilemmas that are not uncommonly encountered in ensuring provision of quality health care.

Autonomy versus Nonmaleficence/Utility

Currently, some QA professionals question the common practice of conducting reviews of patients' medical records for QA studies without patients' knowledge and consent (Maciorowski, 1988). This practice can be viewed as an example of conflict between the principles of autonomy (self-governance) and nonmaleficence (avoiding harmful acts) or utility (providing the greatest good for most persons involved). If ensuring patients' rights and maintaining their autonomy are the major ethical considerations, surely patients should know that their records are being scrutinized for the quality of their care. In fact, most hospitals ask patients to sign documents similar to the University of Nebraska Hospital's Conditions of Admission. This document authorizes release of medical records to the referring physician; to any insurance company, private review agency, third-party payer, or employer, in order to obtain payment for services rendered; to any other health care facilities to which the patient may be transferred; and to employees and students of the medical center. While such documents typically state that patient records may be used in research, they also state that no research will be undertaken without the separate, written, informed consent of the patient.

If patients refuse to sign such documents, can their insurance coverage or their admission to the health care facility be denied? It is possible that patients' signatures on such documents reflect their fear of the consequences of not signing, rather than their acceptance of the terms of agreement. And while the use of medical records for research is addressed in most admission agreements, review of records by QA personnel is not. Ironically, while admonishing health professionals to integrate QA into patient health education programs as an "ethical imperative," Schwartz (1988) fails to address the need for patients to be educated about QA.

With due respect for the recent evolution of QA practice, it should be noted that the risk to patients of having their records reviewed for QA studies is typically perceived to be low. Since the QA professional's role is to prevent harm to patients by reviewing as many records as are needed to provide an adequate sample of data for the aspect of care being studied, obtaining an adequate, representative sample might not be achievable if patients were allowed to refuse. Furthermore, retrospectively obtaining patients' consent would be time consuming at best and impossible at worst and could effectively prevent the achievement of the numbers of QA studies perceived to be necessary to meet the Joint Commission on Accreditation of Healthcare Organizations' (Joint Commission) requirements. Additional problems that could arise if patients' permissions were required before conducting QA studies include whether or not to share results of QA studies with patients as well as the methodological details of who, where, when, and how permission would be obtained.

In spite of the aforementioned problems, discussion of the issue of informed consent for QA studies by QA professionals and hospital administrators would be helpful in identifying the values and beliefs underlying current practices and in sensitizing both groups to the potential risks to clients and health care providers if information is not held in confidence.

Confidentiality versus Nonmaleficence/Utility

According to Siegler (1982), confidentiality has two purposes in health care. First, it acknowledges respect for the privacy of the patient and sensitive information about the patient and decreases the sense of vulnerability and loss that would occur if patients' personal secrets were revealed. Second, it promotes a sense of trust between patient and health care provider, which is essential for accurate diagnosis and treatment. Unfortunately, the traditional idea of confidentiality as closely guarded secrets between patient and health care provider is an outdated concept; Siegler counted as few as 25 and as many as 100 health professionals and administrative personnel (including utilization review and QA reviewers) who had both access to a single patient's record and a legitimate reason to review it. Siegler recommends sharing with patients what confidentiality really means in today's health care system and providing patients with the choice of determining whether the entire record should be available to all who have a need to know, or whether portions should be accessible only to designated persons. Enacting Siegler's recommendations would demonstrate respect for the privacy of personal information in the medical record; however, the difficulties of obtaining valid and reliable data for QA reports, as discussed above, would remain.

Another aspect of confidentiality that has long been a dilemma for QA professionals relates to the anonymity of the health care provider within the context of peer review. QA professionals are in a position to see both positive and negative outcomes of health care and are very much aware of the personal, professional, and legal implications of identifying health care providers whose care is substandard, incompetent, or otherwise hazardous to patient well-being. The principles of nonmaleficence (avoiding harmful acts), as well as professional accountability and responsibility, mandate that health professionals monitor their own practice through peer review. Garrett et al. (1989) state that health professionals whose practice repeatedly threatens the physical, psychological, or medicoeconomic well-being of the patient should be denounced by the appropriate administrative person only after exhausting all other channels of interventions and reporting within the institution.

Clearly, reviewing care provided to clients places the QA professional squarely in the midst of this dilemma. A clear protocol for action steps that the QA professional should take in the event that harmful health care practices come to light is urgently needed, regardless of whether the professional in question is a nurse, physician, or other member of the health care team.

Justice/Fidelity versus Beneficence/Utility

As Davidson (1986, p. 59) states, there is another "controversy brewing, and it centers on the concept of health care rationing." On one hand, Americans believe that health care is a right that human beings deserve by virtue of their humanity (justice); therefore, the health care professional is compelled to provide the best possible care available (beneficence) or, at the very least, the care that the health care professional has promised the client (fidelity). On the other hand, in the real world of limited resources that characterizes today's health care system, the utilitarian position is to provide the best possible care for the greatest number of human beings. This position underlies rationing of health care resources, which currently takes the form of cost/benefit analysis. In today's health care climate, the resources being rationed include facilities (restrictions on construction and renovation), new technologies (determination of which agencies may purchase which pieces of equipment), and personnel (limitations on hiring and training new employees) (Fuchs, 1984).

While Davidson (1986) believes that the utilitarian position is not ethical and not appropriate for discussion within bioethics, the dilemma does exist as a problem of distributive justice versus beneficence, between the obligation to provide the best possible care to society and the obligation to do the same for individuals (Fry, 1985). How, given limited resources in health care, should goods and services be distributed for the benefit of society? Crisham (1986, p. 31) states that while situations of limited resources create dilemmas that are economic in nature, they also create numerous ethical questions, such as who will bear what burden and receive which benefits, or by what principles and procedures can justice be ensured.

The concept of rationing in health care, while not a new one, is becoming evident in QA. Current Joint Commission standards for accreditation require that all major clinical functions of nursing services/departments be monitored and evaluated (Joint Commission, 1989a). This requirement is interpreted to mean that QA professionals should focus their limited resources of time, personnel, and budget on the most important aspects of care or service. Specific variables (indicators) then must be identified for the important aspects of care that are of high volume (occur frequently or affect large numbers), high risk (place patients at serious risk if not provided correctly; show that care provided is not indicated or that indicated care is not provided), or problem prone (have tended in the past to produce problems for staff or patients) (Joint Commission, 1989b). Given this frame of reference, QA time, energy, and resources are being rationed: given to those aspects of care that are high volume, high risk, or problem prone.

The argument can be made that resources are too scarce for QA professionals to monitor *all* high-volume, high-risk, problem-prone areas. Thus rationing is necessary, even if some patient care areas suffer in the end (i.e., those not selected for QA study). Others argue that rationing of QA services compromises patient needs or health problems of populations that do not typically receive QA monitoring because they are minorities in health care facilities, such as the homeless, poor, and elderly.

The selection of areas of care that receive QA monitoring (and those that do not) constitutes an ethical dilemma because of the conflict between the principles of utility (QA monitoring should be provided to the greatest number of patients or patient problems) and justice (limited QA resources should be distributed equitably among deserving groups). Should all patients have an equal chance for QA monitoring? Or should monitoring be selective, focusing only on select groups or problem areas? This dilemma must be squarely faced, without hiding behind the goal of eliminating waste or reducing cost while avoiding the potential consequences rationing of QA resources can bring.

Clearly, the aspects of care and the subsequent indicators selected for QA monitors should be carefully determined by staff nurses, managers, QA professionals, and administrators. The underlying values and motives used in selecting the important aspects/indicators should be clearly identified and articulated. For example, the question arises in regard to whose values are being represented by addressing the aspect of "intravenous medication administration." Is this a value expressed by accrediting agencies, risk management personnel, physicians, nurses, or patients? Is the motive behind this monitor to reduce liability due to adverse patient outcomes, to improve staff compliance with intravenous therapy policies, or to monitor a particular group of patients because the monitors routinely show excellent staff performance?

As the above example shows, QA professionals must recognize whose values, motives, and outcomes QA activities address. Being aware of the reasons for selection of monitors should be helpful in identifying and beginning to resolve the ethical dilemmas surfacing in QA. Knowledgeable, equitable, and logical decisions can then be made, and QA professionals can develop plans for monitoring care and practice that best utilize limited resources while minimizing bias and gaps in the areas of care selected for evaluation.

RESOURCES FOR IDENTIFYING AND RESOLVING ETHICAL DILEMMAS

While there are no simple answers to the ethical dilemmas emerging in QA, a variety of resources are available for assistance in the articulation and resolution of dilemmas. These include personal resources, professional resources, and institutional and other resources.

Personal resources for dealing with ethical dilemmas in QA include QA professionals at local and regional levels, whose expertise can be brought to bear in validating that a particular dilemma exists and in sharing actions taken, if any, to resolve it. Networking at professional QA-related meetings and publication of effective actions plans in newsletters and professional journals specific to QA can be effective in promoting dialogue among QA professionals about dilemmas they are experiencing.

A variety of professional and institutional resources are available to nurses who are grappling with ethical dilemmas in QA, as in other areas of nursing practice. These documents include the American Nurses' Association's (ANA's) (1976) code and the International Council of Nurses' code of ethics (cited in Jameton, 1984, pp. 299–300), as well as ANA's and other specialty groups' standards of practice. The state's nurse practice act and the QA professional's employing institution's standards of practice may also be helpful in identifying expectations for ethical behavior and outlining the scope of nursing's ethical accountability (Blake, 1981). In addition, articles and texts are available that further address ethical decision-making models (Benjamin & Curtis, 1981; Crisham, 1986; Fleetwood, 1989) from the theoretical positions of philosophy and biomedical ethics. As Bernal and Bush (1985) indicate, if nurses are strongly grounded in ethical theory and decision making, they will be better able to defend action plans based on ethical principles and will be able to assert that some values are more important to pursue than others.

Unfortunately, each of the above resources may be limited in its application to specific ethical dilemmas in QA. Codes, standards, and philosophical principles tend to be written in general, abstract language that may be ambiguous and vague. Furthermore, it has recently been suggested that traditional models of ethical theories and principles may not be as compatible with nursing's history and philosophical traditions of caring as another framework might be, such as Gilligan's (1982) ethic of care, which focuses on responsiveness to others and maintaining relationships (Cooper, 1989; Nokes, 1989). Therefore, nurses struggling to articulate and resolve ethical dilemmas in QA may need to avail themselves of additional resources, such as the agency's multidisciplinary ethics committee and consultants with expertise in a variety of ethical frameworks. This does not mean that the QA professional is a passive recipient of ultimate knowledge from an expert in resolving the identified dilemmas; rather, the nurse is an active participant in discussing the dilemmas and searching for sound action plans with other concerned individuals.

IMPLICATIONS AND CONCLUSION

The authors of this chapter believe that if the emerging ethical dilemmas in QA are to be effectively addressed, rational dialogue must occur at a variety of levels within health care organizations, and between health care practitioners and educators of relevant disciplines. Currently, as Joint Commission requirements for health care organization accreditation move QA programs away from retrospective record reviews and toward multidisciplinary concurrent monitors of patient outcomes, discussions of the ways in which QA programs should be implemented are often characterized by anxiety, confusion, and frustration. Anxiety naturally arises from the ongoing process of accreditation and the awareness of the enormous impact that loss of accreditation would have for the organization in terms of economic survival and maintenance of status in the community. Confusion occurs as a result of attempting to understand what the Joint Commission really expects from nursing, medicine, agency administration, allied health professionals, medical records, and other groups/services involved in

QA. Frustration results when the various disciplines attempt to communicate their beliefs about QA to one another, since each group approaches the subject of QA from a different and deeply embedded value-laden perspective.

A few examples should serve to illustrate the variety of approaches held by some of the disciplines involved. Physicians frequently view the quality of their care in terms of morbidity and mortality rates within their particular diagnosis-related groups (DRGs) and strive to maintain these rates at levels consistent with regional or national levels. In contrast, nurses tend to be concerned more holistically with patient outcomes that indicate that safety, comfort, physiological and psychosocial needs have been met; these categories cut across many DRGs. Agency administrators are concerned with providing quality health care at reasonable cost and about implementing efficient and cost-effective QA programs that comply with the expectations of accrediting bodies. Because these differing approaches are so deeply held and reflect the inherent "worth" of each group's expertise, it is small wonder that more heat than light is frequently generated by multidisciplinary discussions of what QA is about.

What can be done to minimize the interdisciplinary conflict and maximize successful resolution of the dilemmas? Davis (1982) recommends that first it is essential to create a climate within the health care organization in which open dialogue can occur. Each group needs to clarify and examine its own values and learn methods of rationally exploring ethical dilemmas while avoiding overly emotional responses. Davis presents three formats of "ethics rounds" for discussing ethical dilemmas; while the dilemmas she has in mind address patient care situations, the format of ethics rounds has merit for discussing ethical dilemmas in QA. Ethics rounds consist of organized discussions of specific dilemmas, led by a group facilitator who is skilled in group leadership and knowledgeable about ethical theories and principles. The goal of such discussions is to examine the dilemma and to discuss options for resolving it that are based on ethical principles instead of personal/professional values. In QA, these discussions can begin with identifying important aspects of care to be monitored, identifying underlying and conflicting values of the various constituent groups in the QA program, and identifying ethical dilemmas as they emerge, such as those identified in this chapter.

Successful articulation and resolution of ethical dilemmas in QA also requires active involvement of QA professionals in health policy formulation, both within the organization and without the organization at local, state, and national levels (Young, 1987). This involvement begins with participating at the local level in determining policies that affect the operationalization of QA programs and progresses to regional and national discussion of such issues as access to health care, standards of practice, distribution of resources, the right to health and health care (Sietsema & Spradley, 1987), and where the responsibility lies to see that health care is provided to which groups (Benoliel & Packard, 1986).

Another avenue of addressing ethical dilemmas and clarifying the value systems underlying the various disciplines involved in QA is educating the professionals involved. Health care administrators and QA professionals must be informed about standards and expectations of external review organizations as well as the ethical principles that can illuminate the ethical dilemmas that are emerging. Medical records personnel should be informed about the different orientations to QA taken by medicine, nursing, administration, utilization review, and other relevant groups, and the implications of these orientations for their work in QA. Agency staff (nursing, medicine, allied health) should be made aware of the values underlying their selection of important aspects of care to monitor, as well as the ethical implications of their choices. Curricula in schools and colleges that prepare health care practitioners should include content on biomedical ethics, ethical decision making and conflict resolution, and appropriate methods of addressing ethical dilemmas within the context of professional role enactment (Benoliel, 1983; Fromer, 1982; Huckabay, 1986; Thompson & Thompson, 1989).

Beyond staff development and formal educational processes of education, awareness of ethical dilemmas in QA can be promoted by workshops and seminars at local, state, and national QA conferences. Such workshops and seminars can be conducted to examine ethical dilemmas and initiate dialogue between QA professionals. In addition, research is needed to answer such questions as, What is the prevalence of ethical concerns in nursing QA? What actions are being taken to address such ethical concerns? What impact, if any, do conflicting interdisciplinary values on the part of health care providers have on patient outcomes?

Clearly, without increasing awareness of the ethical dilemmas emerging in QA via dialogue, educational processes, and dissemination of research results, the current tensions between all of the parties involved in QA will continue to exist. The approach taken in this chapter is one of open discussion of values and application of sound ethical principles to the debate, as QA professionals continue to refine their practice and execute their mission: monitoring the quality and appropriateness of patient care.

REFERENCES

American Nurses' Association. (1976). *Code for nurses with interpretive statements.* Kansas City, MO: Author.

Beauchamp, T.L., & Childress, J.F. (1979). *Principles of biomedical ethics.* New York: Oxford University Press.

Benjamin, M., & Curtis, J. (1981). *Ethics in nursing.* New York: Oxford University Press.

Benoliel, J.Q. (1983). Ethics in nursing practice and education. *Nursing Outlook, 31,* 210–215.

Benoliel, J.Q., & Packard, N.J. (1986). Nurses and health policy. *Nursing Administration Quarterly, 10,* 1–14.

Bernal, E.W., & Bush, E.G. (1985). Values clarification: A critique. *Journal of Nursing Education, 24,* 174–175.

Blake, B.L.K. (1981). Quality assurance: An ethical responsibility. *Supervisor Nurse, 12*, 32, 37–38.

Cooper, M.C. (1988). Covenantal relationships: Grounding for the nursing ethic. *Advances in Nursing Science, 10*, 48–59.

Cooper, M.C. (1989). Gilligan's different voice: A perspective for nursing. *Journal of Professional Nursing, 5*, 10–16.

Crisham, P. (1986). Ethics, economics, and quality. *Journal of Nursing Quality Assurance, 1*, 26–35.

Davidson, L.A. (1986). Health care rationing: Ethical reflections. *Nursing Administration Quarterly, 10*, 59–61.

Davis, A.J. (1982). Helping your staff address ethical dilemmas. *Journal of Nursing Administration, 12*, 9–13.

Fleetwood, J. (1989). Solving bioethical dilemmas: A practical approach. *Nursing 89, 3*, 63–64.

Fromer, M.J. (1982). Solving ethical dilemmas in nursing practice. *Topics in Clinical Nursing, 4*, 15–21.

Fry, S.T. (1985). Individual vs. aggregate good: Ethical tension in nursing practice. *International Journal of Nursing Studies, 22*, 303–310.

Fuchs, V.R. (1984). The "rationing" of medical care. *The New England Journal of Medicine, 311*, 1572–1573.

Garrett, T.M., Baillie, H.W., Garrett, R.M. (1989). *Health care ethics: Principles and problems*. Englewood Cliffs, NJ: Prentice-Hall.

Gilligan, C. (1982). *In a different voice: Psychological theory and women's development*. Cambridge, MA: Harvard University Press.

Huckabay, L.M.D. (1986). Ethical-moral issues in nursing practice and decision making. *Nursing Administration Quarterly, 10*, 61–67.

Jameton, A. (1984). *Nursing practice: The ethical issues*. Englewood Cliffs, NJ: Prentice-Hall.

Joint Commission on Accreditation of Health Care Organizations. (1989a). *Accreditation manual for hospitals*. Chicago: Author.

Joint Commission on Accreditation of Health Care Organizations. (1989b). *Update on nursing services monitoring and evaluation*. Chicago: Author.

Maciorowski, L.F. (1988). Quality assurance data: Whose information is it anyway? *Journal of Nursing Quality Assurance, 2*, 18–24.

Maurice, S., & Warrick, L. (1977). Ethics and morals in nursing. *MCN, The American Journal of Maternal-Child Nursing, 2*, 343–347.

Nokes, K.M. (1989). Rethinking moral reasoning theory. *Image, 21*, 172–175.

Purtilo, R.B., & Cassel, C.K. (1981). *Ethical dimensions in the health care professions*. Philadelphia: WB Saunders.

Thompson, J.E., & Thompson, H.O. (1989). Teaching ethics to nursing students. *Nursing Outlook, 37*, 84–88.

Schwartz, R. (1988). Quality assurance—afterthought or integrated approach. *Patient Education and Counseling, 12*, 185–187.

Siegler, M. (1982). Confidentiality in medicine—a decrepit concept. *The New England Journal of Medicine, 307*, 1519–1520.

Sietsema, M.R., & Spradley, B.W. (1987). Ethics and administrative decision making. *Journal of Nursing Administration, 17*, 28–32.

Young, S.W. (1987). The nurse manager: Clarifying ethical issues in professional role responsibility. *Pediatric Nursing, 13*, 430–432.

SUGGESTED READINGS

Applebaum, P.S., Roth, L.H., & Detre, T. (1984). Researcher's access to patient records: An analysis of the ethical problems. *Clinical Research, 32*, 399–403.

Brubaker, K.M. (1987). Credentialing of medical staff: The nursing department's role. *Nursing Management, 18*, 45–46.

Davis, A.J. (1985). Informed consent: How much information is enough? *Nursing Outlook, 33*, 40–42.

Eriksen, L.R. (1987). Patient satisfaction: An indicator of nursing care quality? *Nursing Management, 18*, 31–35.

Fiesta, J. (1988). Nurses' duty to disclose. *Nursing Management, 19*, 30–32.

Fowler, M.D. (1986). The role of the clinical ethicist. *Heart & Lung, 15*, 318–319.

Fowler, M.D., & Levine-Arif, J. (1987). *Ethics at the bedside: A source book for the critical care nurse.* Philadelphia: JB Lippincott.

Fry, S.T. (1989). Toward a theory of nursing ethics. *Advances in Nursing Science, 1*, 9–22.

Gilligan, C., Ward, J.V., & Taylor, J.M. (Eds.). (1988). *Mapping the moral domain: A contribution of women's thinking to psychological theory and education.* Cambridge, MA: Harvard University Press.

Kittay, E.G., & Meyers, D.T. (Eds.). (1987). *Women and moral theory.* Totowa, NJ: Rowman & Littlefield.

Kravitz, M. (1985). Informed consent: Must ethical responsibility conflict with professional conduct? *Nursing Management, 16*, 34A–B, 34D, 34F–H.

Packard, J.S., & Ferrara, M. (1988). In search of the moral foundation of nursing. *Advances in Nursing Science, 10*, 60–71.

Tribulski, J.A. (1987). Staff development: Practice ethics. *The Journal of Continuing Education in Nursing, 18*, 15–16.

Wilson-Barnett, J. (1986). Ethical dilemmas in nursing. *Journal of Medical Ethics, 12*, 123–126, 135.

10

Interdisciplinary Quality Assurance: Issues in Collaboration

Diane Fay Puta, MS, RN, Director, Medical Staff Services and Quality Management, Sinai Samaritan Medical Center, Milwaukee, Wisconsin

The current health care environment includes care delivery that involves multiple disciplines with both independent and overlapping practices and responsibilities. Because of the multidisciplinary nature of much of today's health care, collaborative interdisciplinary quality assurance (QA) approaches are necessary in order to ensure comprehensive evaluation of care. Successful collaboration among professions in quality assurance activities requires the presence of key interpersonal characteristics and skills applied within interactions influenced by the dynamics and politics of organizational group processes. The inability of interdisciplinary QA interactions to achieve collaborative results can often be traced to inattention to these factors. Several approaches exist that can be used to support positive group/organizational dynamics and aid in achieving successful collaboration in QA activities in today's clinical settings. This chapter will further define collaborative interdisciplinary quality assurance, address the political and interpersonal dimensions that can create barriers to effective collaboration, and discuss approaches for constructive handling of the issues involved in collaboration.

Interdisciplinary Aspects of Health Care

Research in the literature documents the positive impact of interdisciplinary care. A study carried out at the George Washington University School of Medicine, in Washington, D.C., found differences in the mortality rates of intensive care units that "appeared to relate to the interaction and communication between physicians and nurses" (Knaus, Draper, Wagner, & Zimmerman, 1986, p. 416). The study evaluated patient outcomes in intensive care units at several major medical centers.

Today's health care technologies and patient acuity levels are evolving new professional/practitioner roles that often overlap or create new interaction patterns that rely on shared or joint responsibilities in order to efficiently yet effectively manage the care of patient populations (Puta, 1989). Many of today's new treatment modalities and technologies are highly complex, requiring specialized levels of skill and knowledge. This makes it difficult for any one practitioner to be able to independently manage the applications of these modalities and technologies in the care of specific patient populations. As a result, new professional/practitioner roles are evolving that require interprofessional collaboration in order to meet the care needs of patients being treated with the new technologies. Such interprofessional application of treatment modalities and technologies also requires interdisciplinary review of the quality of these applications.

The continuing reduction in mortality from major illnesses has expanded the lifespan of individuals. At the same time, chronic diseases have increased. Patients who become ill often have multiple coexisting conditions that make management of their care more complex, requiring the interaction of a variety of specialists and professionals to treat the whole patient. These professionals need to also collaborate in reviewing the quality of the services provided through their interactive care of these patients.

FACTORS THAT PROMOTE INTERDISCIPLINARY QA

The increasing emphasis on quality in today's society along with new directions in QA are factors that promote collaborative interdisciplinary QA efforts.

Emphasis on Quality

There is a growing emphasis today on quality in patient care, particularly through demands for quality from consumers, and a focus on quality in new legislative and regulatory requirements.

Demands of Consumers

Public media and the organized efforts of specific special interest groups have focused the attention of health care consumers on quality. The news media have stepped up use of media events to publicize health care provider information, such as the mortality rates released by the Health Care Financing Administration (HCFA). Such media events are one means of responding to growing demands for information that can be used to determine the level of quality of services provided by health care organizations.

The American Association of Retired Persons (AARP) is one organization that has been active in providing information in relation to the quality of health care through such means as its publication *Exchange*. One issue announced the availability of a set of criteria for rating hospitals in the Washington, D.C., area (that could also be applied elsewhere). The criteria for judging quality included such items as absence of complications, improvement in functional ability, and ''a pleasant, comfortable stay'' (AARP, 1987–1988, p. 6).

Legislative Pressures

The Health Care Financing Administration (HCFA) is adding to the increased pressures for quality through continuing expansion of mandates that peer review organizations (PROs) include a review for quality as part of their contractual activities (Puta, 1989, p. 12). Peer review organizations exist under contract with HCFA to carry out review of health care services reimbursed through Medicare. In some states the PROs also review care reimbursed through Medicaid. The review criteria utilized by the PROs are developed by physician members of these organizations. Initial care reviews are carried out by nurse reviewers, with secondary reviews and final judgments regarding appropriateness of services being carried out by physicians.

Originally, the HCFA scope of work contracts with PROs required reviews that focused more on admission and continued stay appropriateness. In the 1986–1988 scope of work contracts for PROs, HCFA mandated use of generic quality screens as part of the reviews performed in acute care settings. Most recently, HCFA is requiring PROs to expand such quality review into the ambulatory care settings ("PROs Must," 1988).

Most of the quality screens being used by PROs at this time do not focus on areas directly related to the care provided by any one professional group but instead address aspects of care where interdisciplinary collaboration is important. For example, some of these screens relate to occurrences such as nosocomial infections and patient falls, while others address discharge planning (Curtis, 1986).

The measures of quality being used by the media, consumer interest groups, and HCFA focus primarily on items that are not specific to an individual health care profession (i.e., no one professional group is entirely responsible for these aspects of care). For this reason, interdisciplinary review and evaluation of data collected by use of these measures (to the extent such data are available) would permit health care professionals to examine how they together contribute to the results.

New Directions in QA

The Joint Commission on Accreditation of Healthcare Organizations (Joint Commission) through its Agenda for Change is setting the course for new directions in QA as we move into the 1990s. These new directions include ongoing monitoring, use of clinical indicators, and a focus on outcomes of patient care.

Focus on Ongoing Monitoring

In 1986 the Joint Commission initiated its Agenda for Change project, "intended to improve the Joint Commission's ability to evaluate health care organizations and stimulate greater attention to the quality of patient care" (Joint Commission, 1988, p. 13). A major part of this change project is a revision in the accreditation process. The key change is a move away from the traditional periodic survey and into a process of ongoing monitoring and evaluation through transmission of information from health care organizations to the Joint Commission for analysis and feedback at regular intervals. It is planned that a significant part of the data transmitted for ongoing monitoring will be data collected relative to clinical, organizational, and managerial performance indicators (Joint Commission, 1988, p. 14).

This concept of ongoing monitoring is not too different from the data collection already being done as part of the HCFA quality screening process. One unanswered question is whether the Joint Commission will permit HCFA to access the data from this ongoing monitoring once it is in place. This question arises out of an announcement that as of July 1, 1989, the Joint Commission would already be giving selected accreditation survey information to HCFA (Joint Commission, 1989).

Outcomes of Patient Care

One of the challenges for quality assurance has always been determining what data elements to select to collect data for quality review/assessment. The publication of mortality data by HCFA refueled the debate over whether outcome measures are the best means of assessing quality of care: "Professional consensus is that outcomes such as mortality rates, even if they are adjusted to reflect the severity of illness among patients served, cannot alone be the basis of conclusions about quality; severity-adjusted outcome data can, however, identify potential quality-of-care problems" (Joint Commission, 1988, p. 15).

As the search for better ways to measure quality of care continues, we can anticipate further emphasis on use of outcome measurement as at least part of future QA activities. The new attention being given to assessing quality through monitoring patient care outcomes is yet another reason for QA to move toward collaborative interdisciplinary activities. Unless there is an immediate, severe complication due to a direct professional intervention, it is difficult to determine the exact contribution of each professional discipline to patient outcomes. In fact, it might be better to look at patient outcomes as the synergistic result of the interactions of various professionals. In this view, interdisciplinary review of patient outcomes becomes a positive means for identifying where professional interactions can be improved to effect a more positive result (i.e., outcome).

MEANING OF "INTERDISCIPLINARY QA"

Collaborative interdisciplinary QA is still a new concept in many clinical settings, although its process is inherent to the multidisciplinary practice long in place in such settings as critical care and psychiatric units. There is a lot of confusion over what interdisciplinary QA is and is not. Interdisciplinary QA exists when more than one professional group is involved in the same monitoring and evaluation process (i.e., reviewing the care of the same patient population). There are two different kinds of interdisciplinary QA processes, those in which the QA activities are carried out separately (without direct, face-to-face interactions) and those in which the activities are carried out through interprofessional planning, review, and actions (using face-to-face meetings).

"Parallel" QA

The term "parallel QA" is used here to describe interdisciplinary QA activities in which more than one profession or discipline is carrying out the same activities at the same time without concurrent, face-to-face interaction between them. For example, a parallel QA activity might involve review of all psychiatric readmissions within 30 days of discharge. Physicians, psychologists, nurses, and social workers might all review these cases. If each of these groups reviews the cases and discusses the findings in separate professional meetings, this is a parallel QA activity, not collaborative interdisciplinary QA.

Other literature uses the label "joint responsibility" for the QA processes referred to in this chapter as parallel QA. According to Kohles and Barry (1989), the joint responsibility process "generally does not require an interactive working relationship between disciplines, and, therefore, the most effective outcomes may not be identified or implemented to improve services" (p. 2).

Peer Review

Interdisciplinary QA is also distinct from peer review. Peer review means review of a professional's care, including judgments, decisions, and management approaches, by another individual or individuals of the same professional and/or clinical background. The exact level of sameness required for professionals to be considered peers depends somewhat on the complexity and level of specialization of the care under review, as well as the intensity of the review. For example, in a general definition of peer, any nurse could be considered the peer of another nurse when identifying who is a peer for review of nursing care. However, if the specific review being conducted is examining the appropriateness of decisions, judgments, and actions taken in nursing management of patients on ventilators, another nurse with this clinical background would be a more appropriately designated peer to conduct an in-depth review than would be a nurse from an ambulatory care setting.

The emphasis on peer review in QA has caused some difficulties in continuing development of collaborative interdisciplinary QA because some professionals claim that all QA is peer review, and therefore only peers can or should be involved in the review of a professional's practice.

In fact, while peer review is a significant part of QA, it is still only *one* part. Peer review comes into the QA process when questions are raised that require judgments or assessments to be made about how an individual professional managed an aspect of patient care. This usually comes up when a more intensive evaluation of monitoring data is undertaken. At such a point, delegation of the intense evaluation to professional peer(s) is appropriate.

Some professionals use the peer review concept to try to eliminate interdisciplinary review because of concerns about having "outsiders" become aware of their profession's areas for improvement, or because they do not want to be identified as the source of quality problems. These concerns have evolved from some of the past misuses of QA, in which QA was seen as more of a "snooper-vision" activity, used to "get" people. In addition, the current litigious climate surrounding health care, with increased media attention to malpractice suits, has understandably made some professional groups, particularly physicians, sensitive to having problems identified with their practice brought to the attention of others.

It is important, then, that peer review aspects be separated from multidisciplinary QA processes, in order to protect the confidentiality of such review, to ensure that peer review is truly carried out by peers, and to enable multidisciplinary QA to stay focused on collaborative efforts to improve patient care.

Collaborative Interdisciplinary QA

Collaborative interdisciplinary QA involves the face-to-face interaction of a variety of professional groups in QA activities in order to assess how the combined participation of these groups in patient care supports the progress of patients and the outcomes of care, and to identify where improvements could be made through better professional interaction that would result in better patient care. Kohles and Barry (1989) describe this collaborative process as "a mechanism for personnel from different disciplines to create a relationship that fosters an understanding of the unique skills and knowledge each discipline contributes to patient care. . . .

The uniqueness of each discipline is preserved in this process, and the liaison relationship supports effective quality outcomes'' (p. 1).

Many examples of collaborative interdisciplinary QA are available in the literature. Barmann and Domask (1989) describe interdisciplinary QA collaboration in their article on a multidisciplinary approach to ensuring quality of care for diabetic patients. The particular collaboration they describe involved interdisciplinary collaboration of nursing, physicians, and laboratory personnel to accomplish implementation of QA mechanisms in order to initiate bedside glucose monitoring. According to Barmann and Domask, when the findings from the QA mechanisms substantiated the accuracy of bedside monitoring, this "reinforced the confidence of laboratory, medical, and nursing staff in their ability to provide a multidisciplinary approach to quality care for the diabetic client" (p. 25).

BENEFITS OF INTERDISCIPLINARY COLLABORATIVE QA

The collaboration of professions in QA activities can have many positive results, including early recognition and resolution of problems and improvements in the understanding of, respect for, and working together of professions.

Early Recognition and Resolution of Problems

The collaboration of professionals in the ongoing review and evaluation of the quality of patient care can aid in early recognition and resolution of problems. Rowe and Jackson (1989) describe how concurrent, collaborative interdisciplinary QA helped identify and enable staff to take action to resolve the early beginnings of a complication in a critical care unit at the Montana Deaconess Medical Center. A concurrent review process revealed a slight increase in patients needing surgical repairs for femoral artery access sites. The findings from this review were discussed at an interdisciplinary meeting. Nurses and physicians were able to simultaneously implement actions and engaged the pharmacy to participate as well. A decrease in the problem was reported following implementation of the actions of these professional groups.

Improvements in Interprofessional Relations

Some of the positive effects of collaborative interdisciplinary QA are increased understanding and respect between professional groups, as well as an improvement in their ability to work together. Kohles and Barry (1989) reported that a collaborative QA process involving laboratory and nursing personnel resulted in interprofessional communications that were "more respectful and harmonious" (p. 10).

KEY ELEMENTS OF COLLABORATIVE INTERDISCIPLINARY QA

Putting people from different disciplines together into a combined QA committee or meeting does not in and of itself guarantee that a collaborative QA process will result. In order for interdisciplinary QA to be collaborative, several elements need to be present within the individuals involved in the interaction processes. These elements include mutual trust, open communication, effective communication skills, clinical competence, responsibility/accountability, and assertiveness.

Mutual Trust

Mutual trust is essential because it is only on the basis of such trust that disciplines will be willing to be honest and open in the discussion and evauation of findings from the monitoring of quality. Mutual trust is one characteristic associated with nurse-physician collaboration in the literature (Alt-White, Charns, & Strayer, 1983).

No interactive relationship can develop until mutual trust exists (Johnson, 1972, p. 43). Such trust is important in QA discussions to ensure that individuals will listen to what is said without becoming hostile to those who present the findings or those who question the implications of what is presented. Johnson defines trust as an individual's choice to be open when this could result in positive or negative consequences, with the consequences being dependent on the behavior of others (p. 45).

Communication and Communication Skills

Alt-White et al. (1983) report that "the organizational development literature has repeatedly identified the communication process in a given work setting as being another influential factor in determining the extent of collaboration" (p. 11). Their own research further demonstrated a positive relationship between communication and interdisciplinary collaboration (p. 14).

Open Communication

Open communication is essential to interdisciplinary QA so that objective exploration can be made of the findings from monitoring and quality review activities. Open communication requires the prerequisite presence of mutual trust. Open communication means that professionals are willing to share their interpretations of what the monitoring findings and analysis seem to be indicating, ask questions of one another, identify areas for improvement or further evaluation, and suggest action strategies for initiating improvements.

Open communication also involves disclosing how one is reacting to and feeling about what takes place in the interaction process. This openness requires self-awareness and self-acceptance to prevent feelings and reactions from being hidden and preventing development of mutual trust (Johnson, 1972, p. 3).

Effective Communication Skills

A variety of individual communication skills are also important in developing collaborative interdisciplinary QA. These include the use of constructive feedback and listening skills.

Use of constructive feedback in collaborative interdisciplinary QA communications includes giving and asking for feedback. Frequently the discussions in QA interactions become personalized to either an individual or a profession. One way to depersonalize these discussions is to keep communications as objective as possible. In presenting information, the speaker could use only actually observable data (e.g., what was recorded or observed) and avoid mixing interpretations into the presentation. When analyzing findings, distinctions would be made between interpretations and actual data. If findings lead to unclear interpretations, a suggestion could be made to collect additional objective data to aid the evaluation process. The accuracy of communication can be improved by checking to make sure that the message being sent is the same as the message being received. One way to do this is for the sender of the message to verify that "his or her words are used in the same sense that they will be understood by the recipients" (Kuhn & Beam, 1982, p. 168). Requesting feedback on communications is another way to ensure that a message was understood. Unsolicited feedback, such as is provided by nonverbal cues (i.e., facial expressions indicating confusion or grimaces that might indicate the message was received negatively) is also useful. Another way to improve the accuracy of communications is to use redundancy in communications, such as by giving an example of what is being said or through use of multiple messages (Kuhn & Beam, 1982).

Johnson (1972) points out that failures in communications between individuals or groups usually occur because of a gap between the sender and receiver, "created by emotional and social sources of noise. People, for example, are often so preoccupied that they just do not listen to what others are saying" (p. 64).

Effective listening is critical to communication and the development of collaborative interactions. Johnson (1972) describes one barrier to effective listening as our "natural tendency . . . to judge, evaluate, approve, or disapprove of the statements made by the sender" (p. 75). One technique to avoid judging the sender's statements and develop more effective communication is to use paraphrases or what Johnson labels an "understanding response": "a response that indicates the receiver's intent is to respond only to ask the sender whether the receiver correctly understands what the sender is saying, how the sender feels about the problem, and how the sender sees the problem" (p. 125).

Another barrier to effective listening and communication is selective perception—the tendency to listen to and interpret only parts of what is heard rather than the entire message of the sender. Johnson (1972) points out that communication is so complex that it is impossible to attend to all the verbal and nonverbal aspects of a message (p. 78). Thus the receiver of a message selects what aspects of a message to attend to. The receiver is also selective in what his or her perceptions are relative to the aspects of the message attended to. Receivers of messages focus attention and perception on those aspects of a message that are consistent with their expectations, needs, wants, desires, opinions, attitudes, and beliefs, while misperceiving or even ignoring those aspects of the message that are opposite to their expectations, needs, wants, desires, opinions, attitudes, and beliefs (Johnson, 1972, pp. 78–79).

One way to overcome selective perception is to keep the interpretation of a message tentative until one is able to confirm it with the sender, and to make this confirmation prior to responding to the message (Johnson, 1972, p. 79). The use of feedback is one mechanism for clarifying the interpretation of a message. Such feedback might entail an exact repeat of the words used, then a rephrasing or restatement of what was said in order to indicate the meaning of the words that came across. Johnson (1972) points out that "when paraphrasing is skillfully done, the receiver is able to achieve the sender's frame of reference in regard to the message" (p. 75).

Clinical Competence

Clinical competence means that the individual professional has demonstrated the technical skills and judgment necessary to provide appropriate, effective patient care within the clinical setting in which QA activities are being carried out. Clinical competence is essential to collaborative interdisciplinary QA because it forms one of the bases on which mutual trust develops. As Devereux (1981) states, "No physician can be expected to accept the judgment of or share decisions with a nurse if he has no confidence in her knowledge, skills, or judgment" (p. 32). Professionals are more likely to trust those they recognize as clinically competent to be able to provide meaningful insights into the causes of quality-related problems and to identify appropriate actions to take to resolve problems.

Responsibility/Accountability

Responsibility and accountability are also essential to collaborative interdisciplinary QA. Devereux (1981) identifies willingness to assume clinical responsibility as "one of the pillars of collaborative efforts between doctors and nurses" (p. 38). Individuals who are willing to take responsibility and accept accountability for their own and their profession's role, contributions, and actions (both commissions and omissions) in patient care delivery will contribute to development of an environment of mutual trust and open communication in which quality issues can be discussed and acted on.

Assertiveness

Assertiveness is important in the development of collaborative interdisciplinary QA to ensure that all participating disciplines adequately contribute input to the selection of important aspects of care to be monitored, the review and evaluation of findings, and identification of areas for improvement and planning of corrective actions. Assertiveness as used here means the willingness to communicate one's point of view, even if it may be a minority opinion, and to do so in a manner that is conducive to constructive discussion (i.e., without being aggressive, brash, offensive, demeaning, or accusatory). But assertiveness in collaboration also has to be tempered with cooperation: "Collaboration has a high degree of both assertiveness and cooperativeness, in contrast to modes in which one may yield completely to the other's concerns, may strive to satisfy one's own concerns with no regard for others, or may compromise some important concerns" (Weiss & Davis, 1985, p. 299).

ORGANIZATIONAL GROUPINGS, POLITICS, AND COLLABORATIVE QA

According to Bacharach and Lawler (1982), "survival in an organization is a political act" (p. 1). Because health care professional groups function within organizations, the survival and success of collaborative interdisciplinary QA is influenced by the dynamics of organizational politics.

Organizational Groupings

One major part of the organizational political dynamics affecting collaborative interdisciplinary QA is that of organizational groupings. Bacharach and Lawler (1982) identify three kinds of groups that participate in organizational politics: work groups, interest groups and coalitions (p. 8). They contend that organizational politics is dominated by the politics of these groups, particularly interest groups and coalitions.

Work Groups

Work groups are individuals brought together on the basis of "departmental work activity, or differences prescribed by the organizational hierarchy" (Bacharach & Lawler, 1982, p. 8). Examples of work groups are the staff who work the evening shift on a clinical unit, the registered nurses who work in the critical care unit, or those individuals who fill the position of unit secretary.

Interest Groups

All organizations are "networks of interest groups, whether professional groupings, work groups, or other divisions" (Bacharach & Lawler, 1982, p. 79). Interest groups are individuals brought together through an awareness "of the commonality of their goals and the commonality of their fate beyond simply their interdependence with regard to the conduct of work" (Bacharach & Lawler, 1982, p. 8). Part of the organization's politics involves interest groups seeking to pursue their goals and influence decisions relative to their group. An example of an interest group would be the existence of a professional nurse council or committee, whose members may include the work or professional groupings of clinical nurse specialists, nurse managers, and staff nurses, when such a council or committee exists to unite its members in a commitment to and execution of goals to further the profession of nursing and nursing practice within an institutional setting.

In a QA program, an example of an interest group might be the formation of an inpatient nursing QA council or committee, which would be composed of the work/professional groupings of nurses from the medical surgical units, critical care units and so on. It may also include representation of such groupings as clinical nurse specialists, nurse managers, and staff nurses.

Coalitions

Coalitions are groupings of interest groups "committed to achieving a common goal" (Bacharach & Lawler, 1982, p. 8). Coalitions seeking to influence organizational decisions create another major dimension of organizational politics. Part of the struggle in organizational politics is for interest groups to decide whether to pursue their goals and influence decisions on their own or through coalitions. An example of a coalition might be a multidisciplinary psychiatry QA committee with membership that includes psychiatrists (both private practitioners and faculty), psychologists, nurses, social workers, rehabilitation therapists, and the like, who in turn also represent a variety of programs/services such as drug and alcohol, adolescent and geropsychiatry.

Bargaining Processes in Organizations

Bacharach and Lawler (1982) define bargaining as "the give-and-take that occurs when two or more interdependent parties experience a conflict of interest. . . . Bargaining is the action component of conflict. . . . Resolution of the current issue or problem may also affect future bargaining and bear on the long-term maintenance of good relations" (p. 108). Conflicts are likely to happen in interdisciplinary QA interactions due to the involvement of individuals and subgroups with a variety of interests. Such conflicts of interest can be worked through to further support collaboration through use of integrative bargaining and constructive communication.

Integrative Bargaining

Integrative bargaining involves joint problem solving, so that final resolution of problems benefits all parties (Bacharach & Lawler, 1982, p. 110). According to Weiss and Davis (1985), collaboration uses integrative bargaining because it "involves attempts to find integrative solutions where both parties' concerns are recognized and important concerns are not compromised" (pp. 299).

In interdisciplinary QA, integrative methods might be used when conflict situations arise in trying to take action relative to problems identified, particularly if the conflicts result in polarization. For example, in evaluating problems with stays in a critical care unit, the QA group may agree that some stays are not appropriate in length or admission, and that something needs to be done. But some group members may object to having a single physician make the determination that particular patients do not need to be in the unit. Other members may object to having nurses identify patients that might not belong in the unit.

Using integrative methods, the group members would identify the various reservations relative to the key solutions, then pool their insights, goals, and values to arrive at a resolution that is acceptable to all, without compromising any party's major concerns. In the example used here, the physician members may have reservations about loss of referrals if they have to make the determination about appropriateness of stays. The nurse members may anticipate objections from other physicians if nurses have to identify patients who do not belong in the unit. The resolution might be to develop specific, written criteria for appropriateness of admission/continued stay that are distributed to the medical staff prior to implementation, then are used by the designated physician and nurses to flag patients ready for discharge (or inappropriate for admission). The written criteria then becomes the vehicle for identifying patients, rather than an individual physician or nurse.

Communication and Bargaining

The role of communication becomes critical in the bargaining process used by organizational groupings in conflict situations. Bacharach and Lawler (1982) describe the complexity of communication in organizational conflict situations: "Research indicates that the mere opportunity to communicate does not have a consistent effect on conflict resolution. . . . Overall, it is the content of the communication, not the opportunity to communicate, that is critical" (pp. 114–115).

An example of this in interdisciplinary QA might be a conflict that arises due to physicians' objecting to nurses raising quality of care concerns. Calling a meeting of the physicians and nurses in and of itself will not resolve the conflict. Rather, the content of the discussion at such a meeting is critical to ensure an integrative resolution to the situation. This means exploring the goals, values, and reservations of participants, using this information to point out that the common goal *is* quality of care, then pooling the insights of the participants to arrive at strategies for how quality concerns can be raised without this coming across as nursing judging physician practice.

Such a conflict resolution meeting also would require attention to and use of constructive feedback, and the listening and communication skills cited earlier in this chapter.

GROUP DYNAMICS AND COLLABORATION

Because most interdisciplinary QA activities are carried out in groups, group dynamics influence the extent to which such activities are successful in being collaborative. Group dynamics also create a number of interaction issues that can be barriers to collaboration. These include group membership, group size, meeting dynamics, and group leadership issues.

Group Membership Issues

Group membership issues center on the determination of who will be group members. Membership determination includes decisions about the qualifications and selection of group members. Constructive handling of membership determination issues can help promote collaborative interactions in a group.

Membership Determination

The selection of members for interdisciplinary QA committees is critical as a first step in determining the potential for collaboration. Unfortunately, the ability of individuals to contribute to positive, collaborative interactions (e.g., through demonstration of the characteristics and skills cited earlier) is rarely considered when committee membership is decided. Instead, committee membership is more likely to be determined by organizational position, as a reward, or as a punishment. Examples of organizational experiences might include appointing an individual who actively participates on another committee, thinking that this will automatically ensure his or her active participation on the QA committee; rewarding a practitioner who admits several patients to the institution or performs several procedures by giving him or her an appointment to a committee; or appointing to a committee a person who is not very active in contributing to the organization, in an effort to get additional participation by this individual.

When group membership is decided only on the basis of organizational position, as a reward, or to get someone to do something, this action sets up the group for conflicts of interest and probably little if any collaboration.

Often membership on committees, including interdisciplinary QA committees, is determined by appointment processes. These appointments are sometimes made by individuals who are not very familiar with the interaction characteristics and skills of the individuals being appointed, the requirements essential for collaborative interaction of committee members in interdisciplinary QA activities, or the functions of the committees to which the appointments are being made.

Mechanisms for Constructive Handling of Group Membership Issues

One of the best mechanisms for constructive prevention of group membership issues is to change the way in which membership on committees is handled. The characteristics and skills cited earlier might be used in determining group membership, along with an individual's interest in, commitment to, and knowledge of QA, QA processes, the patient care population(s), and the specific practice/care issues to be addressed by the committee.

Another approach to group membership that might assist in interdisciplinary collaboration involves nomination and selection of a profession's committee representatives by the clinical members being represented. This would mean that members of the professional group (e.g., social service, occupational therapy, nursing, physicians) would nominate the candidates and possibly vote to elect those professionals they wanted to represent them on a committee. There is a caveat with this approach: It can be destructive rather than constructive to collaboration if it is not set up in a manner to ensure consideration of the characteristics and skills cited earlier, or if the motivations in the selection process are political rather than a desire to be represented by the individual most likely to contribute to collaborative QA interactions.

Group Size Issues

Another area that presents problems in interdisciplinary QA is that of group size. Group size issues arise out of representation needs and quorum requirements. Group size also influences the ability of the group to accomplish anything.

Representation Needs

One of the major group size issues is that of representation. Often it is felt that all professional subgroups must be represented by members from their respective subgroups—for example, only a social worker in a specific area can represent social work in that area, only a physician in a specific section of a clinical department can represent that section. As a result of these representation needs, interdisciplinary committees tend to swell to enormous numbers. For a critical care interdisciplinary QA committee, for example, membership may include the manager of each unit (to represent the direct line management), the nursing director, the nursing vice president, plus staff nurses from each unit (to represent the direct caregivers), surgeons, internists, pulmonary medicine physicians, pulmonary services staff and/or management, anesthesiologist, and others. This may result in a committee with a membership of 20 or more individuals, which may not be functional or practical.

Quorum Norms

Another area of group size issues is that of quorum norms. Frequently quorum norms are set up to require at least a 50% attendance of voting members in order for any business to be carried out (Robert, 1970). As committee size increases, the difficulty in attaining quorum norms also increases.

Factors To Consider in Addressing Group Size Issues

In trying to set up effective groups for collaborative interdisciplinary QA, it is important to balance representation of all multidisciplinary aspects of care with maintaining a small enough group size to ensure adequate attendance for quorum purposes and to enable the group to be effective in getting work accomplished.

Mechanisms for Constructive Handling of Group Size Issues

One mechanism for handling representation issues might be to use ad hoc members to represent areas that might not need to be involved in every discussion, yet that the group wants to have available for input periodically. The ad hoc members might be invited to attend at designated intervals, with fixed agenda items to ensure their attendance is utilized, or they might be invited as agenda items requiring their input arise.

Another mechanism for handling representation might be to utilize one member to represent more than one group. For example, on a psychiatric interdisciplinary QA committee, a nurse might represent nursing as well as one of the clinical care programs.

Subgroups of the main group might also be used to ensure adequate representation without making the size of the main group too unwieldy. For example, if the group is a critical care QA committee covering several critical care units, each unit might have its own unit-specific interdisciplinary subgroup to put together representation material for the main committee, yet be represented on the main committee by one member of the subgroup.

Meeting Dynamics

Meeting dynamics, including the politics of interpersonal relationships, group decision making, and handling of conflict, also influence the ability of interdisciplinary QA groups to be collaborative.

Meeting Dynamics Issues

Some of the main meeting dynamics issues focus on the content of meetings, attendance and participation, the ability of a group to accomplish work, and group decision making.

Experience has shown that part of the politics of organizational meetings is their use to accomplish informal agendas of members. There are also the problems of other agenda items coming up that weren't on the order of business (or that aren't even the domain of the particular meeting at which they were raised). At other times responses to agenda items come out of members' feelings about other concurrent organizational issues. Thus what may be seen as a controversial item becomes a major conflict item.

Getting people to routinely attend meetings to ensure continuity of business and getting people to actually participate constructively in meetings are other problems not uncommon in interdisciplinary QA meetings. Along with these problems, there are the people who always arrive late, always leave early, or never show up at all. Sometimes absences from meetings are due to people's being given memberships on several committees, leaving them with a significant time investment, or even an attendance conflict due to meetings that occur at the same time.

Some groups or committees can continually meet without any output to show for their existence. At times a group can have more work to do than can be accomplished within the time frame of scheduled meetings. Other problems can occur when it is time to get the group to make a decision. Sometimes decisions are made by a small subgroup because no one else in the group is willing to speak against them.

Mechanisms for Handling Meeting Dynamics Issues

Several mechanisms can be used to effectively handle meeting dynamics issues. One is the use of agendas, established and distributed far enough in advance to enable members to come prepared to act on items. The agenda should list the business items to be covered at the next meeting and be accompanied by preparatory materials, if appropriate. An even more effective use of an agenda is to word it in such a way that meeting participants know what action will be expected relative to each item (e.g., "Vote on," "Discuss," "Receive information on," etc.). At the meeting, the agenda can be used to steer members back to the group's work when outside issues are brought up.

Meeting norms can be used effectively to prevent or resolve some group dynamics issues, if set up prior to the first meeting of a group. These norms might define what the quorum will be, set up mechanisms for making decisions, identify start and ending times for meetings, and define behavioral expectations of group members (e.g., members will arrive prepared to discuss agenda items; meetings will always start on time and end on time, with a designated length of time preset).

Attendance and participation issues can be addressed in other ways besides through use of group norms. As a courtesy gesture, the chairman of the committee might contact members with poor attendance to determine reasons. This is particularly important to enable those members with legitimate reasons for absences to be able to express these (e.g., schedule conflicts) and to look at alternatives, including replacement on the committee, before the nonattendance becomes an issue to be dealt with in a disciplinary manner.

Attendance and participation in meetings could also be made part of the individual's annual performance (or reappointment) evaluation. To be effective, the evaluation needs to focus on the nature of the participation and not just physical presence at meetings. Pre-established performance standards for committee participation would aid in making such a performance evaluation an objective process. Performance standards for committee participation could be built around the interaction characteristics and skills cited earlier, as well as each committee's own group norms.

If meeting business proves too laborious for the time constraints of members, ad hoc task groups might be set up to handle aspects of the business, then report back to the main group for final action. This would enable the group to keep meetings within a reasonable time frame yet still accomplish something. One often overlooked, but successful mechanism for ensuring effective meeting processes is to initiate new members into the group through use of an orientation process that outlines the group's functions, authority, and norms. This could be done through a face-to-face meeting with the committee chairman or another committee member, or through use of a self-learning packet or audiovisual program.

Another mechanism for making meetings more effective is to use a meeting review or processing technique. This involves assessing the dynamics of the group, using a pre-established tool such as the Meeting Assessment Scale presented by William Martin (1980). This scale "was designed to help uncover possible dysfunctions in regular or semi-regular meetings held by a defined work group. It consists of a list of 30 group and individual behaviors commonly exhibited during the course of meetings" (p. 23). The behaviors assessed with the scale fall into the following categories: structure (e.g., use of an agenda, sense of purpose, clarity of meeting rules), influence (e.g., participation in discussions/decisions), problem solving (e.g., agreement on what the issues are, handling of issues), openness (e.g., willingness to be critical versus personal attacks), and follow-through (e.g., actions are implemented once decisions are made) (Martin, 1980, p. 23).

A tool such as this can be helpful in trouble shooting the dynamics of group meetings that don't seem to be going anywhere or that seem ineffective. For example, use of such a tool might help the group discover that the reason the group is not getting anywhere is because of structure problems: lack of a clear delineation of what the group is supposed to do and how it is to be done. Or the group may discover that nothing gets done due to poor follow-through, because it is not clear who is responsible to take action, or what was to be done.

If use of such a tool is too sensitive for the group members, the group might invite a neutral, objective outsider to attend group meetings and complete the assessment, then provide the group (or the chairman) with feedback.

Group decision making can be another source of conflict in interdisciplinary QA committees. Veninga (1984) cites three possible group decision problem areas: "premature decisions, individual domination, and disruptive conflicts" (p. 44).

Premature decisions occur when enough time is not spent in the decision-making process. Premature decisions can be avoided if group members continually ask themselves and one another if sufficient information is available to make an effective decision. Sometimes premature decisions are made due to time constraints or because group members don't want to sort through all the data available. In these instances, an interim action might be agreed on, with further agreement to collect additional information in order to reassess the action and make a long-term decision.

Domination of a group's decisions by one or two individuals may cause some group members to withdraw from the group or others to respond in an aggressive manner. A skillful group leader or member can prevent domination by making sure that all members have a chance to participate in decisions: "The success of group decision making is contingent upon a perception that everyone in the room has a chance to speak, to be heard, and to be taken seriously. When that perception is present, group members will share their ideas and, once a decision has evolved, will tend to support it" (Veninga, 1984, p. 45).

Group conflicts in a decision-making process can be constructively handled by using the integrative bargaining process described earlier. It is important that whatever approaches are used in group decision making, no attempt is made to eliminate or prevent any or all disagreements, because "disagreements are also a strength, providing that individuals are willing to learn from one another. It is through disagreements that new ideas are born and old ideas are examined" (Veninga, 1984, p. 45).

Group Leadership

One of the overall issues related to group leadership is the selection of the leader. Often individuals become group leaders by appointment, because of activity (e.g., number of admissions, if a physician), by virtue of position (e.g., being the unit manager, or chair of another committee), or because of membership in some other group.

Selection of leaders for a collaborative interdisciplinary QA group is just as important as determining group membership in order to enable successful collaboration to occur. Ideally, the selection of group leaders will involve assessment of their knowledge, skills, goals, and values relative to QA, and their knowledge of the patient population and patient care issues to be addressed. The leader selection also needs to include consideration of the individual's ability to communicate effectively, handle conflict constructively, and manage group dynamics.

Often neglect in the selection or appointment of group leaders can lead to further issues, including designation of a group leader who is ineffective—that is, who is incapable of leading the group. An ineffective group leader in turn can precipitate numerous problems with group dynamics, such as poor meeting attendance, and inability to get things done.

Mechanisms for Handling Group Leadership Issues

One mechanism for effective selection of group leaders is to thoroughly screen potential group leaders prior to the final selection (or appointment) process. This might be done through a self-administered survey tool that includes questions to identify goals, values, and knowledge. Use of the survey tool might also be combined with an interview and/or observation of the individual in actual group interactions, or by asking others about the individual's group leadership.

In order to prevent (or address) the issue of an ineffective leader, a "consultant" might be identified as a resource to the group leader, to assist him or her in working with the process dynamics. The consultant might sit in on meetings, then meet with the leader afterward to provide constructive feedback on what went well and where areas exist for improvement in how the leader functioned and how the group responded.

PEER REVIEW, CONFIDENTIALITY, AND COLLABORATIVE QA

As was mentioned earlier, peer review and concerns over the confidentiality of QA information have often been barriers to successful collaborative interdisciplinary QA. This can be avoided through separating peer review functions from collaborative QA and by using mechanisms for protecting the confidentiality of QA data by elimination of identifiers or use of protected codes, so that group members do not know who the individuals are behind the data being reviewed and evaluated.

As was stated earlier, peer review functions do not belong within interdisciplinary QA. When the review and evaluation of data leads to identification of a single practitioner as a source of a potential problem, the final evaluation of that practitioner's performance relative to professional standards belongs to a peer group, particularly if the problem requires determination of the appropriateness of the practitioner's judgments or level of clinical knowledge.

One way to ensure that peer review is appropriately supported is to set up a norm that individual practitioner patterns will be referred to the respective professional group for final evaluation and actions.

CONCLUSION

Collaborative interdisciplinary QA is both a challenge and a necessity in the current health care environment, in order to ensure the most effective outcomes for patients while acknowledging the interdisciplinary aspects of patient care. Collaboration can become a reality amid organizational groups and political dynamics through attention to interaction characteristics and skills and through implementation of a variety of group process techniques.

REFERENCES

Alt-White, A.C., Charns, M., & Strayer, R. (1983). Personal, organizational and managerial factors related to nurse-physician collaboration. *Nursing Administration Quarterly*, 8–18.

American Association of Retired Persons. (1987–1988). Rating hospitals. *Exchange, 2*, Dec.–Jan., 6.

Bacharach, S.B., & Lawler, E.J. (1982). *Power and politics in organizations*. San Francisco: Jossey-Bass.

Barmann, K.A., & Domask, M.E. (1989). A multidisciplinary approach: Assuring quality of care for the diabetic client. *Journal of Nursing Quality Assurance, 3*, 19–25.

Curtis, M.R. (1986). Current scope of work guidelines for peer review organizations (PROs). *Journal of Quality Assurance, 8*, 11–12.

Devereux, P.M. (1981). Nurse/physician collaboration: Nursing practice considerations. *Journal of Nursing Administration, 11*, 37–39.

Joint Commission on Accreditation of Healthcare Organizations. (1988). *Guide to Quality Assurance*. Chicago, IL: Author.

Joint Commission on Accreditation of Healthcare Organizations. (1989). Joint Commission to share specified survey information with government agencies. *Joint Commission Perspectives, 9*, 5–6.

Johnson, D.W. (1972). *Reaching out. Interpersonal effectiveness and self-actualization*. Englewood Cliffs, NJ: Prentice-Hall.

Knaus, W., Draper, E.A., Wagner, D.P., & Zimmerman, J.E. (1986). An evaluation of outcome from intensive care in major medical centers. *Annals of Internal Medicine, 104*, 410–418.

Kohles, M.K., & Barry, P.L. (1989). Clinical laboratory and nursing personnel: Collaboration in improving patient care. *Journal of Nursing Quality Assurance, 3*, 1–10.

Kuhn, A., & Beam, R.D. (1982). *The logic of organization*. San Francisco: Jossey-Bass.

Martin, W. (1980). When your meetings aren't meeting their objectives. *Training/HRD, 17*, 21, 23, 24, 27.

PROs must begin nonacute care reviews, despite reservations. (1988). *Hospital Peer Review, 13*, 73–79.

Puta, D.F. (1989). Nurse-physician collaboration toward quality. *Journal of Nursing Quality Assurance, 3*, 11–18.

Robert, S.C. (1970). *Robert's rules of order*. Newly revised. Glenview: Scott, Foresman & Co.

Rowe, M.A., & Jackson, J.D. (1989). Multidisciplinary QA in a critical care unit. *Journal of Nursing Quality Assurance, 3*, 35–40.

Veninga, R.L. (1984). Benefits and costs of group meetings. *Journal of Nursing Administration, 14*, 42–46.

Weiss, S.J., & Davis, H.P. (1985). Validity and reliability of the collaborative practice scales. *Nursing Research, 34*, 299–305.

11

The Nursing Quality Assurance Coordinator: An Evolving Role

Mina Acquaye, BSN, MPH, RN, Nursing Quality Assurance Coordinator, South Community Hospital, Oklahoma City, Oklahoma

Patricia Schroeder, MSN, RN, Nursing Quality Consultant, Quality Care Concepts, Inc., Thiensville, Wisconsin

The creation of specialized positions in health care has traditionally occurred in response to the impact of environmental changes. Positions such as the skin care clinician, for example, have been created in many agencies to meet the growing needs of consumers and the constraints imposed by regulatory agencies such as Medicare. Intravenous therapy teams were developed to meet the increasing demand of intravenous therapy and to ensure that a consistent quality of care was being rendered. In an attempt to combat nosocomial infections, the role of the infection control practitioner was created in the 1950s in England. In the early sixties, North America responded by creating an infection control nurse (Wenzel, 1982). The continued rise in health care costs has caused health care agencies to reexamine care delivery with an eye toward delivering it in an economical yet safe manner. The position of utilization review coordinator has been created in order to monitor this.

Advanced roles in nursing, such as clinical nurse specialist (CNS), have evolved to meet the needs of patients and nursing staff in providing care to patients with complex needs. Added to these specialized and advanced roles in the nursing department is the role of the nursing quality assurance coordinator (NQAC).

EXTERNAL AND INTERNAL FACTORS IN THE DEVELOPMENT OF THE NQAC ROLE

Like all the other processes of life, health care organizations have transformed to keep abreast of environmental constraints that are being continually placed on them. Perhaps the most drastic change in health care has been due to the passage of the Tax Equity and Fiscal Responsibility Act (TEFRA) of 1982. This led to the creation of prospective payment systems (PPS) for Medicare patients (Beyers, 1988). These changes shook the financial cornerstones of the health care systems.

To balance the drastic changes imposed by PPS and still maintain a safe environment for patients, quality assurance (QA) processes needed to be intensified to help ensure safe, comprehensive, yet cost-effective care.

Agencies such as the Joint Commission on the Accreditation of Healthcare Organizations (Joint Commission) have also intensified their efforts to ensure that health care facilities deliver optimal care. Their standards for QA under their Agenda for Change call for continual improvement of the quality of nursing care (Joint Commission, 1990).

Other reasons why QA has gained momentum in recent years include an increase in consumers' awareness of what constitutes good-quality care. Since nurses are the largest group of health care professionals in hospitals and are more in contact with patients than any other group of employees, patients often judge the quality of an institution by the quality of the nursing care they receive there (Miller Bader, 1988).

Internal forces are also promoting the importance of QA programs. Hospital administrators have discovered that quality care and service are not just the "right" thing to provide but are cost-effective and can be used as marketing tools to attract more patients and physicians. These administrators also realize that nursing has a great part to play in enhancing an organization's quality efforts. In a survey conducted for hospitals by a consulting firm, 663 chief executive officers rated nursing care over care provided by all other health professionals as the highest indicator of what they consider to evidence quality care (Koska, 1989). As a result, administrators are facilitating and expecting constant improvement in these realms.

Many external and internal factors have caused health care agencies to re-examine their QA programs and to continually strive for improvement in them. Nurses have been pioneers in the QA arena and have created the role of the NQAC to meet the growing needs of QA. Ten years ago, the NQAC position was uncommon. Today, NQACs have become an important part of the nursing department (Masters, Acquaye, MacRobert, & Schmele, 1990).

THE ROLE OF THE NQAC

It is important to distinguish the differences between the role of the NQAC and that of the QA coordinator (QAC). While a variety of titles may be used, typically the QAC is responsible for conducting medical staff and hospital-wide QA. This person also serves as a leader of the organization's overall QA program. In smaller agencies, the QAC may also have responsibility for the QA program in the nursing department. The NQAC, however, is responsible for coordinating the QA activities for the agency's nursing department. The role of NQAC may be a full-time position, a part-time position, or an added duty for a director of nursing

(American Nurses' Association [ANA], 1982). Regardless of the hours allocated to the role, the NQAC has been described as the focal point around which a nursing department's QA activity revolves (Masters et al., 1990).

Today's NQACs can be considered marketers, promoters, and educators of QA in an institution's nursing department. As marketers and promoters, they must continually develop strategies for selling QA in a manner that is appealing and attractive enough for staff to buy into the program. As educators, they must ensure that the entire staff and the nursing management team understand the process and are informed of the latest trends in and expectations for QA. To accomplish this, the NQAC conducts presentations, distributes current literature, or coordinates periodic QA workshops.

Marketer, promoter, and educator are but a few of the multiple roles the NQAC assumes. Rowland and Rowland (1988) utilize the ANA's guide for nursing QA to describe nine roles of the NQAC: coordinator, planner, data specialist, advisor, support person, overseer, recorder, evaluator, and communicator.

As a coordinator, the NQAC serves as a channel of QA information and facilitator of communication from unit to unit and from the nursing QA committee to staff nurses. The NQAC coordinates many nursing QA functions, serves as liaison between nursing QA and hospital-wide QA, and can also serve as a facilitator or cofacilitator of joint studies between nursing and ancillary departments. As a data specialist, the NQAC may assist in data collection, analysis, and reporting. He or she is responsible for developing mechanisms to track problems until resolved.

As a planner, the NQAC maintains and revises the nursing QA plan. The NQAC serves as a facilitator for developing unit-specific QA plans and monitoring activity calendars. He or she is responsible for the development of nursing QA committee agendas and for assisting in planning and prioritizing patient care problems in nursing.

The NQAC functions as an advisor by assisting in data collection, tool development, and formulating changes needed to correct and improve patient outcomes. He or she also plays a major role in recommending the format for the development of standards of care and practice, in a collaborative manner that keeps the NQAC from becoming the author of these standards (White & Baker, 1981). The NQAC also serves as a support person by functioning as the resource person for QA in nursing. Nurse managers may utilize the NQAC as an expert to assist in improving a facet of QA on their unit. Unit QA chairpersons may seek assistance from the NQAC in developing a unit-specific agenda for meetings. As an overseer, the NQAC is responsible for developing a mechanism for facilitating the overall monitoring activities on each nursing unit and ensuring that areas that are not systematically monitoring patient care are advised to do so. The NQAC is also responsible for making sure that nurses on all units are using the appropriate QA process.

As a recorder, the NQAC is responsible for documenting all QA activities and continually ensuring the confidentiality of QA data. Data must also be stored in an easily retrievable manner for the appropriate agencies or personnel who might request them. As an evaluator, the NQAC is responsible for assisting units in testing the reliability and validity of data collection instruments and for ensuring that the nursing department QA program improves patient care and outcomes. The NQAC then makes recommendations to improve the program if it is found to be deficient in accomplishing its goals. Finally, the NQAC serves as a communicator by publicizing QA activities and findings and acting as spokesperson for the nursing department QA program in hospital-wide committees such as infection control, safety, and hospital QA.

These multiple roles serve as a frame of reference for understanding the kinds of skills needed by a NQAC. The many roles also offer an opportunity for growth and creativity for the NQAC.

Role Development

Masters et al. (1990) describe the development of the NQAC on a continuum of stages, from being a novice to being "well seasoned." They portray the frustrations and tunnel vision of the novice NQAC, but also emphasize the opportunities for growth and challenge associated with the role. They emphasize the tremendous amount of self-learning and self-development associated with the role and describe strategies for developing the role. Their description of the seasoned NQAC paints a picture of a self-confident member of the nursing department who has a great deal to offer in terms of continually fine tuning the QA program. The various dynamics associated with the NQAC make the role challenging and fascinating for those involved in it.

THE NQAC IN CENTRALIZED AND DECENTRALIZED QA PROGRAMS

There are two QA program structures within which NQACs typically function: centralized and decentralized, or unit based.

In centralized programs QA activity is conducted through committees or through computer programs that collect data on the same aspects of care from unit to unit (Schroeder, 1988). In this type of structure there may be one or more QA committees; the NQAC and other staff nurses may collect data also.

The more common structure for conducting QA activities is the decentralized or unit-based (UBQA) program. It involves the functioning of a QA committee on each nursing unit and helps to promote greater staff nurse participation in the process (Schroeder, 1988). The NQAC is the coordinator of the UBQA system. Formella and Schroeder (1984) describe the responsibility of the NQAC in this system as one who helps to motivate, maintain, and keep the system operational. Since the UBQA system also requires that staff make decisions about their practice (Schroeder, 1988), the NQAC must ensure that the concepts and processes involved in QA are well known and understood by staff.

The structures within which NQACs function may not be the same, but their roles and responsibilities do not greatly vary. Either way, the NQAC must strive to facilitate and develop the program.

EDUCATIONAL PREPARATION

While certain advanced roles in nursing, such as the CNS, have had a history of advanced education, the NQAC has not had the same advantage. It is mainly through the school of hard knocks that the NQAC learns the role (Warner, 1985).

Formal Preparation

There are few formal educational programs available to prepare a nurse to become an NQAC. Certain schools offer specialized programs at the master's and doctoral levels. The University of California, San Francisco, for example, offered a program of study designed to prepare graduates for leadership positions in QA. The course work emphasized needs assessment, program planning, implementation, and evaluation of a QA program. The University of Pennsylvania also offered a program on QA. Certain schools of nursing and health-related programs offer courses in QA at the baccalaureate and master's levels, but there is great variation in content. As a result, nurses assuming this position have utilized more informal approaches to learn their role.

Informal Preparation

A study conducted by Hoare, Burns, and Akerlund (1985) suggests that initial preparation for the NQAC role has traditionally occurred through self-study, such as reading books and articles written about QA, attending workshops, networking, and on-the-job training. Learning about the role also occurs through functioning in the role on a day-to-day basis in a way that is best understood by the practitioner. Utilization of a framework such as the nursing process (Masters et al., 1990) can help penetrate the mystery surrounding QA and help the NQAC understand the QA process.

The use of a mentor (or a person who may not necessarily be knowledgeable about QA but is knowledgeable about role development) can assist the NQAC in self-development (Masters et al., 1990). Consultants and/or seasoned NQACs outside one's organization can provide support and guidance to the neophyte NQAC. The NQAC may benefit by using as many of these resources as possible in order to obtain a variety of perspectives. Learning is enhanced as these sources of information are reinforced. Learning must never cease for the NQAC.

Continuing Education

To keep pace with the ever-changing approaches to QA and quality improvement, it is essential for the NQAC to read QA journals and review updated accrediting and regulatory agency manuals. Workshops or seminars can further expand one's knowledge base. Courses in computer applications, basic statistical analysis, the application of change dynamics, and conflict management are useful for the NQAC (Rowland and Rowland, 1988). Self-development courses such as in time management may also help to broaden the NQAC's scope of knowledge. Programs and publications on QA topics used in industries outside of health care can also serve to broaden the NQAC's perspectives. Other industries have been in the forefront of quality management for much longer than health care (Gillem, 1988). Current application of continuous quality improvement and total quality management programs in health care organizations is an example of following the lead of other industries.

Certification

Certification provides another avenue for self-development. Certification has been defined as a mechanism for recognizing competence in a field according to certain standards, and is achieved mainly through testing (del Bueno, 1988). There is little or no evidence, according to del Bueno, to support an assertion that certification makes one professional perform better than his or her colleague. And yet certification continues to be considered a professional hallmark and a method of distinguishing professional competence.

The National Association of Quality Assurance Professionals (NAQAP), a national organization, offers a certification program for those involved in QA (Kibbee, 1988). The content of the certification exam, however, is not specific to nursing. It includes utilization review and other medical staff–related issues and does not include review of some functions that may be major aspects of the NQAC's role. The American Board of Quality Assurance and Utilization Review (ABQAUR, 1990), functioning in conjunction with the American College of

Utilization Review Physicians, also offers certification in QA, but as the name suggests, this certification addresses hospital-wide QA and utilization review. Some nurses raise concerns that despite the need for advanced-level knowledge and skills to carry out the role of the NQAC, there is still no certification program that addresses today's role.

SKILLS NEEDED BY THE NQAC

Kibbee (1988) describes practitioners involved in QA as clinical information specialists who need at least four kinds of skills: technical, managerial, consulting, and interpersonal. While it is important to be a clinical information specialist, the consumers' needs for quality have changed drastically, and their "threshold for quality is continually being raised" (Baker, 1987, p. 27). For this reason, today's NQAC cannot concentrate on clinical issues alone but must further expand his or her skills in determining consumers' needs. The four basic skills outlined by Kibbee will be used as the framework to describe the skills needed by the NQAC.

Technical Skills

Technical skills needed in the NQAC role include the development of valid, reliable, and practical indicators and data collection tools. This could require basic skills in statistics, such as measures of central tendencies. A basic knowledge of computer applications can facilitate the tabulation, tracking, and reporting of QA data in a manner that is easy to understand and interpret and subsequently use.

Excellent communication skills are essential for increasing awareness, stimulating interest in QA issues, and disseminating information about patient outcomes (negative and positive) to staff. Communication must be understood by all, staff and management alike; therefore, the NQAC must possess good writing and verbal communication skills (Schmitt, 1987). Reports must be clear, concise, and easily understood. Terminology should be geared for the group of people being addressed. QA jargon is acceptable if everyone is familiar with it and understands the terms. But if the NQAC is giving a presentation to new nurses or nursing students, for example, terminology that is in plain English must be used. In giving QA information, the NQAC should carry it out in a manner that does not put blame on anyone (Hoernschemeyer, 1989). Oftentimes professionals involved in QA tend to emphasize indicators that are below threshold and do not dwell enough on indicators that have met or exceeded threshold. The skills of the NQAC in giving QA information must be done in a well-grounded manner so that staff do not reject QA and perceive it as a negative activity.

Communication is not one sided; it also implies listening. It means the NQAC must possess or develop the skills for listening and taking in information. Such information may be about quality of care, professional competence, interpersonal politics, or systems issues. It may involve listening to things one doesn't want to hear. Communication is a medium for teamwork and getting people to be action oriented (Hoernschemeyer, 1989). In short, communication skills are essential to the NQAC role.

Managerial Skills

Kibbee (1988) states that NQACs typically engage in the management of themselves, time, and information. An example of managing oneself is the ability to prioritize and focus on issues that are most important to patient outcomes. For the NQAC, time management is essential for such things as meeting deadlines for reports or for spending adequate time on each nursing unit interacting with staff and patients. Because supervision is minimal and the role relatively unstructured, the NQAC must be capable of prioritizing and managing busy work that does not fulfill the goals set for QA.

When managing information, the NQAC must possess the necessary skills to organize, store, process, and easily retrieve QA information. Without good organizational skills, the tremendous amounts of QA data generated can be overwhelming. Without good data management, QA data may not be used to their greatest benefit.

Problem-solving skills are another form of managerial skill needed by the NQAC. In their book *The One Minute Manager*, Blanchard and Johnson (1987) describe a good manager as one who is able to guide staff to solve problems themselves. The NQAC must use his or her problem-solving abilities in a manner that facilitates problem resolution at the unit level by the unit staff.

The NQAC has been described by Prescott (1985) as a facilitator and a catalyst for instituting change. The NQAC may be the one to identify and recommend change but may be limited in his or her capacity to actually implement the changes. For example, if the cause of readmission for a certain group of patients is drug toxicity related to inadequate discharge instructions by staff, the unit must create ways to improve their discharge instructions and evaluate and document patients' comprehension. If increased intravenous therapy site infections are due to lack of compliance with the agency's policies for site care, a change is in order. The NQAC cannot independently make the change, but the NQAC may be able to help the unit staff analyze practice on the unit and the value and applicability of the policy, and so create improvement indirectly.

Consultation Skills

Webster's Twentieth Century Dictionary (1978) defines "consultation" as "the art of conferring with others, giving them information and/or advice about a particular issue, meeting to plan or to decide something."

Like other consultants, the NQAC's role as a consultant can take on several forms. In one instance, the NQAC may engage in problem definition and solution on a particular unit. The NQAC accomplishes this by using clues or probing questions to assist a unit to gain insight into a problem. In so doing the unit diagnoses and treats its own problem (Sedgwick, 1973). Consultation is also done when NQACs offer their expertise in designing a QA study or project or utilize their expert knowledge to help a unit fine tune a facet of the QA program, making sure that the guidelines set for QA are followed.

In other instances, consultative activities carried out by the NQAC could be accomplished in the capacity of change agent or serving as a catalyst to initiate change. In this case NQACs can make use of their change principle knowledge base (Stevens, 1978). Consultation by the NQAC can also be done solely to educate staff about QA and to clarify the gray areas of QA. An example of this would be when a unit manager requests that the NQAC teach new nurses about certain QA principles, concepts, or the QA process itself.

To be successful at consultation, the NQAC must possess excellent consultation skills to carry out the role and must continually seek to learn the dynamics behind consultation (Sedgwick, 1973). Also, the relationship between the NQAC and the consultee must be a good one (Beecroft, 1988). The NQAC must therefore continually seek to maintain good rapport with staff and management. To be a good consultant, the NQAC must keep abreast of changes in the internal environment that influence nursing. Such changes might include new patient populations in the clinical areas. The NQAC could use this information to develop process and outcome indicators for monitoring and evaluation. Changes in the mode of delivery of nursing care, changes in equipment, and changes in practice patterns would likewise be of interest to the NQAC and would be used within the QA program.

To keep up with these internal changes, the NQAC must stay close to practice. One way to accomplish this is to deliver hands-on care periodically, working enough hours to maintain clinical perspectives. This not only keeps one on top of changes in nursing practice in the agency but also provides for close observation of the clinical setting, the clinical performance of others, and their understanding of the QA process. Spending more time on each nursing unit and less time in one's office also helps the NQAC to stay close to practice. Spending time on the units might include organizing focus groups with staff. This could help the NQAC to identify their needs and gives the NQAC an opportunity to establish rapport with staff nurses; they in turn can see the NQAC as one who understands nursing practice and its difficulties. Focus groups can also be held with patients and their families in waiting rooms. One-to-one patient and family interviews can be conducted also. Participating in data collection in the clinical setting also gives the NQAC the ability to stay close to the "real action."

The opportunity for mingling together that the consultation process provides the NQAC and QA members or staff promotes a collaborative relationship between them. As a result, consultation opportunities must always be sought, and NQACs must be flexible enough to respond immediately to units that request consultation.

Interpersonal Skills

The NQAC should also be actively involved in assisting the department of nursing to create "the socio-cultural conditions needed to develop and nurture teamwork, collaboration and personal commitment" to quality (Baker, 1987, p. 27). In order to create such an atmosphere, today's NQAC should possess or develop interpersonal skills, such as supporting and empathizing (Kibbee, 1988).

The NQAC must continually strive to support staff and management in all he or she does. Support should not only be given in the area of QA activities but also in other activities. Activities outside of QA could include exercises such as patient care conferences or discharge planning conferences.

The NQACs role in creating an atmosphere of empathy cannot be overemphasized. They must recognize that people's needs, desires, and abilities need to be taken into consideration as well (Baker, 1987). An empathetic and supportive NQAC is better able to win staff over to QA.

NETWORKING AND THE NQAC

Networking, a source of support and professional growth, is vital in any profession and more so for the NQAC due to the dearth of available formal training. Networking gives the NQAC an opportunity to exchange information and ideas (Kibbee, 1988). The importance of establishing networks outside one's organization cannot be overemphasized. For the seasoned NQAC networking can serve as a source of professional growth, whereas for the novice NQAC it will serve as a means of support (Masters et al., 1990). Networking can be conducted internally and externally.

Internal Networking

The role of the NQAC can be isolated and lonely. NQACs may identify and interact with practitioners in their organization that are at the same professional level, such as CNSs and staff development coordinators. Because these peers are in a position that is not solely or directly related to QA, sharing professional information, strategies, and support must be done in a broad sense. These practitioners can function as colleagues, collaborators, or sounding boards for the NQAC. Opportunities to network with other NQACs must be sought in order to attain a better knowledge base and sense of support.

External Networking

The NQAC may pursue networking locally or nationally. NQAC network members not only share technical information about QA but also function as a forum for unloading the frustration that is associated with noncompliance or lack of support for QA. A great deal can be shared regarding strategies to break the barriers to quality. Discussing the difficulties assists both the new and the seasoned NQAC to realize that some of his or her problems are universal.

Networking can also extend beyond the NQAC group by linking a unit QA committee chairperson with a similar unit in another organization, to facilitate networking at the grass-roots level. An example of this would be linking the leader of one facility's oncology nursing QA committee to the leader of another; specific and valuable information relating to QA in the oncology unit can then be shared.

Hayko and Elrod (1987) describe several advantages to networking. The main purposes behind networking are to provide educational opportunities, support, and sharing of patient care evaluation methods.

The educational needs of network members are assessed so that presentations of teaching programs can be offered by the group members. Network members who attend workshops can also share their knowledge with the group.

The support network members provide one another, according to Hayko and Elrod (1987), may be in the form of providing a forum for discussing problems and concerns without violating the confidentiality of each organization. For example, if an organization is experiencing an increasing rate of urinary tract infections (UTIs), the NQAC of that agency can solicit from the network members ideas on how to deal with the problem. Data on the actual rate of UTIs need not be identified. Sharing of ideas and resources can be an ongoing beneficial process. One example might be the sharing of strategies utilized in generating QA interest in staff and management. Sharing of policies, procedures, standards, and documentation forms can also be done. To prevent reinvention of the wheel, data collection tools can be shared, especially if indicators are common from one institution to the next. If tools are agency specific, it may be easier to adapt them rather than develop a tool from scratch. Tools are particularly valuable if they have been tested for validity and reliability by other agencies and are ready to be applied.

There are some disadvantages to networking too, such as the problem of language barriers and issues of confidentiality and sharing within a competitive environment. Most network members, however, draw largely upon its positives and develop strategies to decrease the disadvantages.

EVALUATION OF THE NQAC

In any role, evaluation can facilitate growth and development (Porter, 1988). Since most NQACs assume their role without any prior training, frequent evaluation, especially during the first year, can serve as a "powerful teacher and motivator" (Wiley, 1988). Ideally, for a neophyte NQAC a formative method of evaluation will be used. This kind of evaluation offers the NQAC a more frequent opportunity to be evaluated, which allows the NQAC to identify strengths and weaknesses sooner than at the end of a designated end point, such as 6 months or 1 year (Nadzam, 1987, Sommerfield & Accola, 1978). By determining areas of needed development sooner, the NQAC can be more timely in personal development.

Evaluating the NQAC is done by using the performance evaluation based on the job description. When the job description is well designed, written in behavioral terms, and describes accountability, it can make evaluation much easier (Morath, 1988). For example, if part of the NQAC's job description is to orient new staff nurses to the concepts of QA, this information can be obtained with the assistance of the staff development department. Or, if the annual evaluation of the QA program is a responsibility of the NQAC, documentation of such activity can be easily retrieved.

In the article "The Clinical Nurse Specialist: Evaluation Issues," Morath (1988) describes mechanisms for evaluating advanced practice nurses, two of which are peer review and self-evaluation. These mechanisms can be utilized for the NQAC as well.

Peer Review

The evaluation of professionals must include peer review (Porter, 1988). Unfortunately, peer review can be a problem if one holds a unique role in an agency. However, unit managers and unit QA facilitators can serve as peers to some point. These people work hand in hand with the NQAC, have insight into QA, and can determine if the NQAC is an effective resource person, consultant, and planner. They are in a sense the closest in understanding the NQAC's role. Those closest to understanding the practitioner's role should be involved in the peer review (Morath, 1988).

The CNS and the nurse educator may also have roles that parallel that of the NQAC in some way, so their input could be beneficial. In addition, some who hold unique roles look to those in similar roles in other agencies for peer feedback and evaluation.

SELF-EVALUATION

Self-evaluation emphasizes that NQACs are accountable and responsible for their own practice (Morath, 1988). To conduct an effective self-evaluation, realistic, clear, measurable goals must be set in advance, in order to give the NQAC some target at which to aim. Goals should be mutually set by the NQAC and other key members of the nursing department, and efforts must be made to ensure that goals are in congruence with organizational and departmental goals for QA.

While the above methods of evaluation can serve as avenues for growth and development of the NQAC, other forms of evaluation must be considered as well. An unsuccessful QA program may not always be a fair reflection of the NQAC's ability, due to the fact that the success of a QA program depends on other factors, such as management and staff commitment. However, the NQAC's ability to promote the program, facilitate development of effective tools that lead to the detection of negative patient outcomes and practice problems, analyze the cause of problems, and spearhead corrective action can in turn give staff the opportunity to become aware of the effectiveness of QA. When staff see the impact that QA has made, they tend to attribute such achievements to the input of the NQAC, and this can serve as a method of evaluating the NQAC.

Using combinations of evaluation systems must be considered when evaluating the NQAC. The importance of feedback regarding the progress or lack of progress in the NQAC role cannot be overemphasized. An effective evaluation can improve the NQAC's ability to function and develop in the role.

CONCLUSION

This chapter has painted a complex picture of the role of today's NQAC. It has portrayed the flexibility and creative opportunities that exist for the NQAC due to the multiple roles that are associated with this position. Health care QA is a growing area, and so is the role of the NQAC. In the future the academic sector must adapt and enhance its curricula to ensure that nurses are educated to assume this role. Health care institutions must also respond by recognizing the NQAC's voice as an important one in an agency's nursing department and for its overall quality efforts.

As QA processes progress and evolve, the role of the NQAC will change as well. Such changes may be reflected in the day-to-day work of the NQAC. Changes might also be reflected in the position the NQAC occupies in the nursing department's hierarchy. The capabilities of the NQAC have not been fully tapped within many of today's nursing departments. The effective NQAC must continue to be empowered with the necessary resources, information, and support to fully realize organizational and personal capabilities.

REFERENCES

American Board of Quality Assurance and Utilization Review Certification Flyer. (1990). Venice, Fla.: Author.

American Nurses' Association & Sutherland Learning Association, Inc. (1982). *Nursing quality assurance management/learning system, guide for nursing quality assurance coordinators and administrators.* Kansas City: American Nurses' Association and Sutherland Learning Association, Inc.

Baker, E.M. (1987, November). The quality professional's role in the new economic age. *Quality Progress*, 20–28.

Beecroft, P.C. (1988). The consultant's image. *Journal of Nursing Administration, 18*, 7–10.

Beyers, M. (1988). Quality: The banner of the 1980's. *Nursing Clinics of North America, 23*, 617–623.

Blanchard, K., & Johnson, S. (1987). *The one minute manager.* New York: Berkley Books.

del Bueno, D. (1988). The promise and reality of certification. *Image: Journal of Nursing Scholarship, 20*, 208–211.

Formella, N.M., & Schroeder, P.S. (1984). The unit-based system. In P.S. Schroeder (Ed.), *Nursing quality assurance: A unit based approach.* Gaithersburg, MD: Aspen Publishers.

Gillem, T.R. (1988). Deming's 14 points and hospital quality: Responding to the consumer's demand for the best value health care. *Journal of Nursing Quality Assurance, 2*, 70–78.

Hayko, D.M., & Elrod, M.E. (1987). A community-wide quality assurance resource group: Benefits in today's environment. *Journal of Nursing Quality Assurance, 2*, 59–64.

Hoare, D.H., Burns, M.A., & Akerlund, K. (1985). The perceived training needs of quality assurance professionals in eight eastern states. *Quality Review Bulletin, 7*, 87–92.

Hoernschemeyer, D. (1989). The four cornerstones of excellence. *Quality Progress*, 37–40.

The Joint Commission on Accreditation of Healthcare Organizations. (1988). *The Joint Commission guide to quality assurance.* Chicago: Author.

The Joint Commission on Accreditation of Healthcare Organizations. (1990). *The Joint Commission 1991 accreditation manual for hospitals.* Chicago: Author.

Kibbee, P. (1988). An emerging professional: The quality assurance nurse. *Journal of Nursing Administration, 18*, 30–33.

Koska, M.T. (1989). Quality . . . thy name is nursing care, CEO's say. *Hospitals, 63*, 32.

Masters, F.K., Acquaye, M., MacRobert, M., & Schmele, J.A. (1990). Role development: The nursing quality assurance coordinator. *Journal of Nursing Quality Assurance, 4*, 51–62.

Miller Bader, M.M. (1988). Nursing care behaviors that predict patient satisfaction. *Journal of Nursing Quality Assurance, 2*, 11–17.

Morath, J. (1988). The clinical nurse specialist: Evaluation issues. *Nursing management, 18*, 72–80.

Nadzam, D.M. (1987). Documentation evaluation system: Streamlining quality of care and personnel evaluations. *Nursing Management, 18*, 62–63.

Porter, A.L. (1988). Assuring quality through staff nurse performance. *Nursing Clinics of North America, 23*, 649–655.

Prescott, A.R. (1985). Quality assurance professionals in the U.S.A. *World Hospitals, 21*, 40–41.

Rowland, H.S., & Rowland, B.L. (1988). *The manual of nursing quality assurance*. Gaithersburg, MD: Aspen Publishers.

Schmitt, A. (1987). What it is like to be a quality assurance manager. *Nursing Life, 7*, 18–19.

Schroeder, P.S. (1988). Directions and dilemmas in nursing quality assurance. *Nursing Clinics of North America, 23*, 657–664.

Sedgwick, R. (1973). The role of the process consultant. *Nursing Outlook, 21*, 773–775.

Sommerfield, D.P., & Accola, K.M. (1978). Evaluating students' performance. *Nursing Outlook, 26*, 432–436.

Stevens, B. (1978). The use of consultants in nursing services. *Journal of Nursing Administration, 3*, 7–15.

Warner, A. (1985). Education for roles and responsibilities in quality assurance. *Quality Review Bulletin, 11*, 78–80.

Wenzel, P.R. (1982). *The handbook of hospital acquired infections*. Boca Raton, FL: CRC Press.

White, J., & Baker, R. (1981). Coordinating a quality assurance program. *Dimensions Health Service, 58*, 43–44.

Wiley, L. (1988). How to do better evaluations with less bother. *Nursing, 88*, 32L–32M.

12

Program Evaluation and Nursing Quality Assurance

Mildred Sawyer-Richards, MPH, RN, Director, *Nursing Quality Assurance,*
St. Luke's Roosevelt Hospital Center, New York, New York

PROGRAM EVALUATION DEFINED

In today's "new" health care environment, legitimate concerns are surfacing regarding the way health care organizations are managed. As health care providers, we find ourselves subjected to ever-increasing scrutiny and calls for accountability from the public, from government, and from the health regulatory agencies. Sheldon and Barrett (1977) describe the effect: "Legislators have shown a greater propensity to regulate health care costs; consumers' expectations are on the rise; community representatives demand to be heard; money is limited, and its use more and more restricted" (p. 77). Health care managers' decision-making practices will in future be closely examined. Michnich, Shortell, and Richardson (1981) agree that management accountability, especially in health care services, may include justification of inaction and actions. One could conclude that a health care program's effectiveness or ineffectiveness will be associated with the system or foundation by which management decisions are made.

Programs are implemented by organizations, and the assessment of organizational performance must account for activities related to organizational survival and growth (Donabedian, 1980, p. 20). Formal program evaluation is viewed by Michnich et al. as an important resource for health care decision making. It is necessary in situations where traditional organizational evaluative capabilities can no longer meet the requirements of the job at hand (Michnich et al., 1981). Program evaluation provides a structured process or mechanism for the QA manager or professional to identify problems interfering with achievement of stated objectives or desired goals. Such awareness provides vital information to be used for the decision making aspect to resolve and/or improve the areas of ineffectiveness. Without the program evaluation component the problem areas would remain. Thus the program would not meet the desired outcome.

Managers of nursing quality assurance (QA) programs have found themselves overwhelmed with the number of QA projects that were due yesterday. Additionally, being a resource and consultant, among many other things, to all levels of nursing can contribute to their losing sight of program needs and priorities. They frequently find themselves working on QA projects that were due last week, while putting out daily fires. Pressures are all around. To counteract such pressures, the program evaluation process can assist with every phase of a program's problem solving needs. For example, when patient care systems are developed by nursing and discussed, the information gained may support and justify the implementation as well as enable a healthy interdepartmental dialogue. This would not be possible without the detailed information gained from the program evaluation process.

Program evaluation has been identified as a set of approaches that can be used to make a value judgment about a program or any of its components, with a view to modifying the program or any of its components (Shortell & Richardson, 1987, p. 8). We could refine this further to define program evaluation as a process of determining the effectiveness of a program in relation to the program's purpose or objectives. By thoroughly applying this process, we will find answers to the questions, What's working? What's not working and why? What changes need to be made to make our program work better and/or improve its effectiveness?

Again, being managers and professional administrators of QA programs, we recognize the importance of demonstrating an effective, comprehensive program. This means we must develop a method of accurately gaining information about program components, especially those with shortcomings that must be improved.

WHY SHOULD WE EVALUATE QA PROGRAMS?

There are several major reasons to evaluate a QA program. First, evaluation supports compliance with the QA standards of the Joint Commission on the Accreditation of Healthcare Organizations (Joint Commssion). From a practical viewpoint, the QA standards of the Joint Commission require an annual appraisal of the QA program. This appraisal is conducted "to identify the scope, purpose, and effectiveness of current activities; to ascertain whether such activities meet all [Joint Commission] requirements for review or evaluation; to identify strengths and weaknesses in the overall QA program; to determine whether duplication in activities, overlap in authority and responsibility, or unnecessary expenditures in staff time and resources exist; and to determine whether expansion, reorganization, or streamlining of the current program is necessary and appropriate" (Shanahan, 1983, p. 29).

Shanahan interprets the standard as being designed to relieve managers of ineffectual evaluation activities and emphasizes that management has an incentive to administer an assessment activity in a systematic and effective manner. She further outlines additional purposes for the standard:

The intent of the standards is to

- allow greater flexibility in quality assurance activities
- encourage innovation and creativity in the evaluation process
- encourage the elimination of duplicative committees, activities and functions
- encourage the coordination of fragmented activities throughout the hospital
- promote systematic and effective evaluation of overall patient care
- encourage communication about the results of evaluation so that improvements in patient care and clinical performance can be assured. (p. 29)

Shanahan suggests ongoing program assessment for whatever tools or methods are employed, even though the standard only requires an annual program evaluation. Program evaluation as a process, she notes, is a "problem-solving" mechanism.

Second, evaluation facilitates the program's growth, integrity, and effectiveness. The ultimate goal of evaluating QA is to determine whether the program is effective in changing nursing practice to improve patient care. This requires a control mechanism to determine a program's effectiveness or ineffectiveness. The information provided from an ongoing program evaluation process can also be viewed and used by the QA manager and administrator as a system of maintaining control. Management actions can be appropriately taken on the basis of such evaluation data.

Smeltzer (1985) recognizes this and supports the evaluation process as a necessary management tool. She states, "Evaluating the effectiveness of a QA program is the most important aspect of planning, implementing and maintaining the integrity of the program"; she further states that "a QA program cannot fulfill its definition of assuring the patient of excellent nursing care unless the program itself is proven effective" (p. 15). In Smeltzer's view, evaluation is the means by which accountability for the effectiveness of the QA program is measured. Evaluation quantifies to what extent the program is successful in improving patient care; special attention is paid to deviations and cost analysis in relationship to expected benefits.

Third, evaluation facilitates the reduction of risk management problems. QA programs exist for the same reasons hospitals exist—to care for patients and ensure that health care professionals fulfill their responsibility to provide safe and appropriate care. Effective problem-solving mechanisms are important to reduce and control potential liability problems for the hospital. There is an increased consumer awareness of the quality of care received. Many consumers who are merely unhappy, not harmed, are now seeking legal redress. As a result, the courts are holding health care professionals liable for providing substandard care. Program evaluation provides important information that can reduce liability risks, as the process utilizes standards of care as measures of practitioners' performance (Culp & Miller, 1985).

Fourth, evaluation directly supports the maintenance of professional values. QA has meaning as it provides a professional framework for nursing administration and other health care providers. When a QA program demonstrates effectiveness, we ensure the entire nursing profession's credibility. Additionally, we maintain two important values, professional autonomy and professional accountability. We meet our obligations to the public and the hospital's administrator and governing board. Most important, we instill greater satisfaction and confidence within our nurses, when they see we regulate our practice. Scott (1983) states, "A hallmark of the autonomous professional organization is that the dominant professional group organizes itself as a professional staff to support and police the performance of its members" (p. 44). We must never forget that it has been a long-sought goal to assert our professional autonomy. Now that we have it, we must never lose sight of our history and struggle.

LITERATURE SUPPORT FOR QA PROGRAM EVALUATION

Program evaluation and its link to QA as a valuable resource tool for decision making has been recognized by the following notable authors. Donabedian (1980, p. 82) in describing the concept of defining quality, emphasizes the importance of a set of activities he calls the "process" of care. Determinants concerning the quality of that process may consist of direct observation or a review of recorded information. He supports the proposition that the most direct route to assessment of the quality of care is an examination of that care via the use of approaches to assessment, as well as an assessment of "structure and outcome." He identifies the relationship between structure and the quality of care as a component of importance in the planning, design, and implementation of systems, specifically those intended to provide professional health services.

Clemenhagen and Champagne (1986, p. 383) note that the concept of the QA system is an important part of the program evaluation process. These authors advise managers or department heads to consider the development of a conceptual evaluation framework. Such a framework is felt to be helpful in terms of understanding the relevance and usefulness of program evaluation activities. They further examine the role program evaluation plays in structuring the general work responsibilities of managers and clinical department heads. Additionally, they describe the two major evaluative activities that managers engage in to carry out their managerial control function: overseeing the provision of services and controlling or regulating activities in accordance with the program's requirements.

The authors suggest that managers define and develop program evaluation criteria to assess program components once they are defined. The evaluative activities can then be focused on prerequisites, implementation, and effects. They also present a "cue" sheet for health care managers to use in evaluating the quality of care.

Wilson (1984, p. 205) states, "Today's nurse-managers are increasingly involved in the development of more efficient and less expensive health care programs." Wilson supports the need for program evaluation and advises nurse-managers to acquire a working knowledge of program evaluation.

Mehnert (1985, p. 127) describes a reassessment process as a necessary management tool to review a hospital's QA program and to systematically re-examine the problems addressed, the methods used to resolve them, the success or failure of these solutions, and the individuals involved. Only then can the QA coordinator determine if the program is comprehensive in scope and identify its successes and failures. The information can then be used as a management tool for setting both short-range and long-range goals. Mehnert describes an innovative form, Program Evaluation Assessment Report (PEAR), which tracks all facets of each problem from identification through resolution. He further states that the frequency of reassessment will depend on the volume of problems handled by the QA coordinator.

CONSIDERATIONS IN EVALUATING QA PROGRAMS

The following list consists of suggested program aspects the author feels, from practical experience, are important for the program evaluation process. The list is provided for QA managers to use and adapt according to their institution and their program needs. The list does not profess to be inclusive and should be used as a resource for indentifying what program aspects to evaluate.

External Requisites

- Does the program meet the requirements of its regulatory agencies (e.g., Joint Commission, state and national government, professional organizations)?
- Have past surveyed deficiencies been corrected? Do you know the status of the deficiencies?

Internal Requisites (Structure, Process, and Outcome)

- Is there a written QA plan? A plan improves the effectiveness and efficiency of the program. It includes clear and measurable objectives and covers the line of authority, coordination, and methods of problem identification for follow-up.

- Is the program efficient? To evaluate efficiency is vital. Efficiency is viewed in terms of the program's cost utilization of mechanisms, activities, staff, and the facility. This information will identify whether the efficiency or inefficiency is due to what's available but not appropriately used, or lacking and needed to meet desired program outcomes. The following factors may be helpful to evaluate efficiency:

1. Is there an experienced and accountable person to coordinate the program?
2. Is there coordination of accountable staff for various QA functions?
3. Are the data organized and easily retrievable?
4. Do QA mechanisms and activities link with other departments in the institution (e.g., Hospital QA)? (This facilitates corrective actions that affect, but may be beyond the control of, nursing.)
5. Is there a risk management data tracking and control system to ensure appropriate follow-up on all identified patient care problems, from the monitoring and evaluation mechanisms in your department to those outside your department (e.g., regulatory survey results, hospital committees)?
6. Is there a system for adequate data gathering? (Sample model size must be appropriate enough to draw a valid conclusion.)
7. Do you schedule QA monitoring and evaluation activities? (Note: A QA calendar that is disseminated to all levels of staff is helpful to remind them of activities; you can color code the calendar for different levels (e.g., management = green, head nurses = yellow, etc.)
8. Do you use other monitoring mechanisms besides the medical record (e.g., observation, interview, staff surveys)?
9. Are various approaches (such as creative workshops, resource meetings, etc.) used to increase understanding and promote the meaningfulness of the QA program? (This is especially helpful for staff nurses.)
10. Have you assessed whether there is any duplication of effort (e.g., committees, monitoring and evaluation)?
11. Are QA reports streamlined and succinct? (Too much information will decrease their utilization.)
12. Is there a communication structure that provides feedback to administration, management, and staff?
13. Does a component of the program reward and acknowledge the contributions of management and staff (e.g., a creative booklet acknowledging improvements in patient care)?
14. Is there evidence of support from nursing administration, management, and nursing staff?

15. Are successful problem-solving methods and strategies shared with other units? (A program evaluation workshop can be used. Units will share accomplishments, areas to improve, and problem-solving methods. To gather together staff from all units greatly improves the meaningfulness of the program, as information is shared.)

- Is the program effective? The program must demonstrate that the desired program outcomes were achieved. Evidence includes demonstration of improved care and maintenance of outcomes.
    1. Are changes and improvements in the nursing department and patient care occurring (behavioral and organizational level)?
    2. Are problems being followed to resolution?
    3. Do the patients, and the patient care services provided, demonstrate evidence of improvement?
    4. Are desired patient outcomes achieved and maintained?
    5. Are monitoring and evaluation activities comprehensive for the scope of services?
    6. Are all major clinical functions for patient groups served by the hospital included with monitoring and evaluation activities?
    7. Are conclusions and recommendations reported to the organization-wide QA program, as specified in the organization's QA plan?

- Does the program provide a cost/benefit analysis? The following should be reviewed:
    1. staff time used for data collection, interpretation, and analysis
    2. the amount of support staff require (secretaries, clerks, administrators)
    3. the need for and use of office equipment and supplies
    4. costs of duplicating reports and QA information
    5. costs for resource materials (books, computer literature searches)
    6. degree of involvement of all levels of staff (at the author's hospital, it was noted that nursing attendants or aides were not involved with monitoring and evaluation activities. The program evaluation process identified this, and units are now using them to monitor, for example, height and weights and to observe skin care via skin care rounds.)

PROGRAM EVALUATION AND RESEARCH

Formal program evaluation frequently is confused with research or the use of scientific methods. Michnich et al. (1981) state that the distinction between formal program evaluation and research has to do not necessarily with the methods employed but rather with the way the results are used. Also, formal program evaluation is designed to supplement real-world decision making, while research adds to the discipline's knowledge. This should clarify that we do not necessarily have to apply the scientific method to make a professional judgment.

TIMING: AN IMPORTANT PROGRAM EVALUATION CONSIDERATION

There are two basic types of formal program evaluations. The first type is *formative,* or implementation, evaluation. This type of evaluation is often used in the early stages of a program's development to assess whether the program is being implemented as it was originally intended, and whether it is in need of revisions. The second type is *summative,* or outcome, evaluation. This is used at the end of a program to review the program's overall impact and efficiency in terms of meeting intended objectives (Schriven, 1967).

From the author's experience, both types should be used to ensure a comprehensive program evaluation process. Formative evaluation allows the necessary ongoing program revisions. Such revisions should be based on information obtained. The summative provides information regarding the effectiveness of the program revisions; thus at the end of the year one can definitely see the program's impact.

TYPES OF EVALUATION MODELS

The D'Costa and Sechrest Model

This model describes (1) an integral relationship between the program administrator, program development, and the evaluation process and (2) the sequential stages of formal program evaluation (Michnich et al., 1981). The model presents the following areas for program assessment review:

1. implementation setting
2. past problems or program improvement aims
3. adequacy of strategic planning, resources available to achieve goals
4. efficiency of resource utilization
5. demonstrated outcomes (unachieved or unintended)
6. value of outcomes in terms of societal impact
7. implementation effectiveness
8. policy changes from which society would benefit

The Zimmer Model

Zimmer's model includes 11 steps that incorporate the findings of evaluation research to include outcome measures of nursing care as a component of the overall evaluation program. Because she uses outcome measures, this model has been highly successful for use in clinical settings. Additionally, she uses nursing peer groups to conduct the evaluation. This model is beneficial for evaluating the outcomes of the nursing care provided to patients (Loveridge, 1983, p. 258).

The Richards Management Model

The Richards Management Model (Figure 12-1) is used by the QA manager and other professionals. It focuses on program outcomes and uses the nurse QA

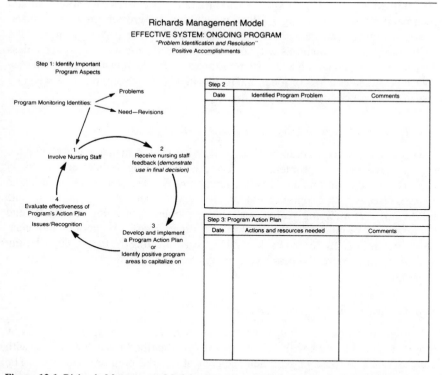

Figure 12-1 Richards Management Model: program evaluation. *Source:* © 1989 Mildred Sawyer-Richards.

administrator and providers of care as integral components of the program's problem-solving process. The power behind a program of excellence is the nursing staff. The author has discovered that this type of commitment and participation is required to support the identified program modifications, to ensure effectiveness. Additionally, this model supports nursing communication at all levels and uses marketing strategies by recognizing program accomplishments. There are three basic steps to the model.

Step 1: Identify Important Program Aspects

QA programs may be different in structure and needs, but there are basic important aspects that can be used as measures for the evaluation process. This step affords a QA manager flexibility in tailoring the evaluation process by focusing on what is really important to evaluate, based on program needs. Program measures from the external commands and internal department needs can be identified for focus (see below). These program aspects, once identified, should become part of an ongoing evaluation activity for greater program control. Program aspects can be viewed as sections, phases, or part of a monitoring activity. Program evaluations will not work as a decision-making resource unless they are part of an ongoing and systematic process. Evaluating a QA program only once a year creates a loss of focus and results in ineffective programs, as well as a loss of program control.

Step 2: Identify Areas of Effectiveness and Ineffectiveness

This step provides structure and focus. It assists the QA manager in isolating the high-priority issues or problems interfering with the program's effectiveness by identifying problems that are (1) affecting a large number of staff and creating an adverse effect on the program's outcome (i.e., perception problems, incomplete follow-up), (2) affecting patient care (i.e., problem not being resolved), and (3) producing problems for the program and nursing staff (i.e., poor communication structure, results not fed back to staff). By controlling the factors contributing to a program's ineffectiveness, we can achieve an effective and comprehensive program.

Step 3: Identify the Program Action Plan

"Program action plan" denotes the action taken by the manager of a QA program. These actions will improve or resolve identified issues interfering with the program's purpose or with achievement of desired program outcomes. The goal is to confirm the program's demonstration that the nursing profession is delivering safe and appropriate care. It answers the question, What needs to be done?

When the need for a program action plan is identified, the QA manager must decide what nursing resources and/or administrative nursing support are necessary to implement modifications. This can greatly facilitate better planning for the change process. This step requires the QA manager to

1. define the possible causes and scope of a problem, in relation to its impact on the program's ineffectiveness (i.e., unrealistic schedule of monitoring and evaluation activities, not enough staff involvement, etc.)
2. make recommendations for change (i.e., change structure of coordination, decrease the schedule of activities)
3. receive valuable information regarding suggestions, from nursing administration and staff who know what will work (This is the most critical information. Listen to valuable information and use it!)

The Richards Management Model is a formative type of evaluation model. Revisions are made, objectives are modified, and program components may be added or deleted. The summative evaluation is used annually with this model to focus on the overall program's impact. This system has been highly successful.

Again, the author recognizes and applauds the vital problem-solving information obtained from all levels of staff. Nursing service in the author's hospital achieved a QA program of excellence because all levels of nursing participated in the evaluation process and were committed to taking appropriate actions when modifications were necessary. This model is simple, practical, and works to bring everyone together with the team philosophy an effective QA program must demonstrate.

TOOLS TO FACILITATE PROGRAM EVALUATION

Evaluation tools can be used to assist the program evaluation process. The author recommends this for the nursing QA program and the unit-based structure.

Summative-Type Tools for the Nursing QA Program in General

As seen in Exhibits 12-1, 12-2, and 12-3, summative evaluation tools assess and provide information regarding three program components:

1. Objectives: Were these met? Not met? Identifies objectives for next year.
2. Effectiveness: What were patient outcomes? Did care improve? Identifies proposed changes to improve effectiveness.
3. Efficiency: Were resources utilized appropriately? Proposes changes for next year.

Exhibit 12-1 Summative-Type Evaluation: Objectives

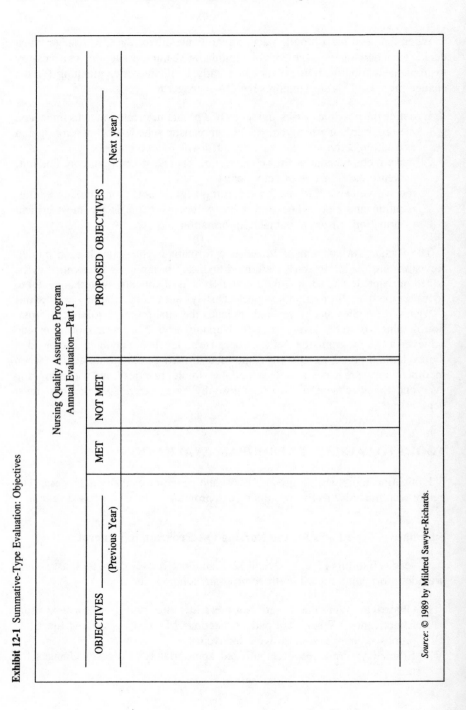

Nursing Quality Assurance Program
Annual Evaluation—Part I

OBJECTIVES _____ (Previous Year)	MET	NOT MET	PROPOSED OBJECTIVES _____ (Next year)

Source: © 1989 by Mildred Sawyer-Richards.

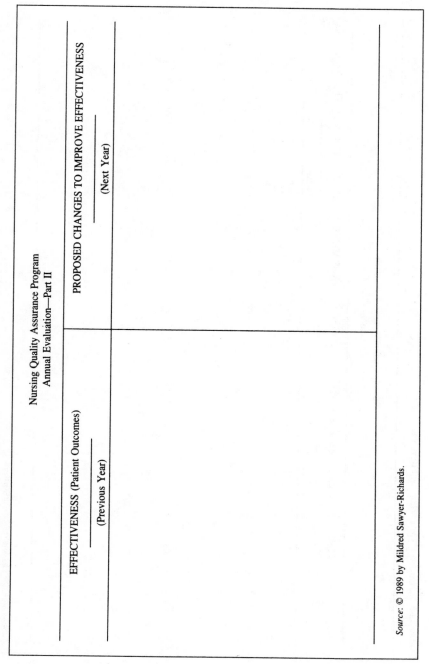

Exhibit 12-2 Summative-Type Evaluation: Effectiveness

Nursing Quality Assurance Program
Annual Evaluation—Part II

PROPOSED CHANGES TO IMPROVE EFFECTIVENESS

(Next Year)

EFFECTIVENESS (Patient Outcomes)

(Previous Year)

Source: © 1989 by Mildred Sawyer-Richards.

Exhibit 12-3 Summative-Type Evaluation: Efficiency

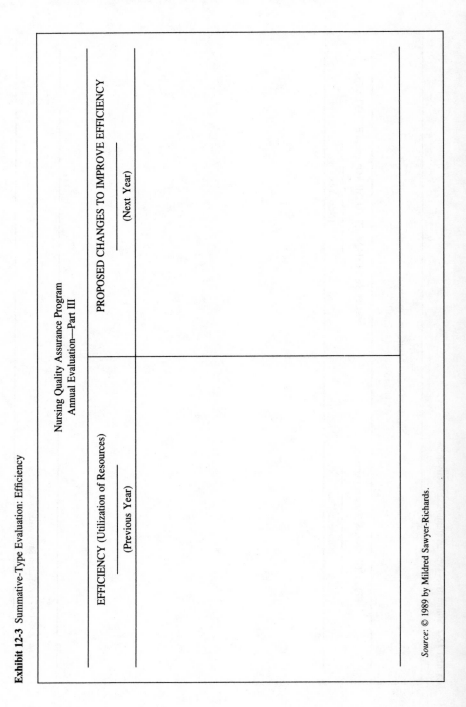

Nursing Quality Assurance Program
Annual Evaluation—Part III

EFFICIENCY (Utilization of Resources)

(Previous Year)

PROPOSED CHANGES TO IMPROVE EFFICIENCY

(Next Year)

Source: © 1989 by Mildred Sawyer-Richards.

Summative-Type Tools for Unit-Based QA Program Annual Evaluations

Exhibits 12-4 and 12-5 are presented to assess three items:

1. important aspects of care, monitoring methods and whether desired patient outcomes were met or not met
2. proposed aspects of care, monitoring methods, and whether additional resources will be needed for the next year
3. effectiveness of care (The unit will identify the changes and/or improvements.)

Program Evaluation Tracking Tool

This tool is part of the Richards Management Model (Exhibit 12-6). However, it can also be used as an ongoing program tracking tool to identify program problems and track their resolution. The author developed this tool from practical experience. It is suggested that the tool be used on a quarterly basis. Quarterly information provides an appropriate time to evaluate and identify an appropriate program action plan. The quarterly time frame further assists in tracking and trending high-volume program problems and ensures a resolution of issues. This provides a control mechanism and structure, the focus for a QA manager and professional.

POTENTIAL BENEFITS OF QA PROGRAM EVALUATION

Hospital Benefits

QA sometimes is seen as creating a problem for health care providers and institutions. But when a department such as nursing can manage an effective program to ensure that quality care is being provided, it creates a marketing edge for the hospital. This increases respect for the nursing administrator and staff. Consequently, it improves relationships with other departments. It also validates the premise that nurses are the "diplomats" for patient care.

The results of program evaluations may be combined to form a basis for health care policy decisions in the organization's structure, to improve patient care services. An effective QA program will demonstrate the institution's effectiveness in caring for its patient population. It will provide evidence of changes from the aggregate of information the program evaluation process provides.

Exhibit 12-4 Nursing QA Annual Unit-Based Program Evaluation, Part 1.

Part 1   Year: _____

List important aspects of care (high volume, high risk, problem prone)	Monitoring methods (i.e., chart, observation)	Desired patient outcomes	
		Met	Not Met

Proposed Aspects of Care (high volume, high risk, problem prone)	Monitoring Methods (i.e., chart, observation)	Will additional resources be needed?

Source: © 1990 Mildred Sawyer-Richards.

Exhibit 12-5 Nursing QA Annual Unit-Based Program Evaluation, Part 2

Part 2   Year: _____

Effectiveness: Has the program resulted in changes and/or improvements with nursing practice and patient care (changes may be completed or in process)?

_____

_____

_____

_____

_____

_____

_____

Efficiency: Has the program made good use of all the resources provided?

_____

_____

_____

Proposed objectives:

_____

_____

_____

Source: © 1990 Mildred Sawyer-Richards.

Nursing Department Benefits

The program evaluation process provides the nursing administrator with improved quality control and a method to evaluate organizational effectiveness, the effect nursing practice has in achieving desired patient outcomes. The program's areas of effectiveness and ineffectiveness are brought to the administrator's attention. The result is resource information helpful in making necessary

Exhibit 12-6 Tracking Tool

Richards Management Model
Tracking Tool—Program Evaluation

Quarterly Report (circle): 1   2   3   4

Date	Program Problem	Cause and Scope	Status (Findings/Action)	Date Resolved

Source: © 1989 Mildred Sawyer-Richards.

organizational changes (i.e., in policies, procedures, committees) to minimize interference with quality patient outcomes. Program evaluation as a process can improve the delivery of patient care, patient care services, and nursing practice.

Unit-Level Benefits

Many authors have recognized the benefits of having patient caregivers address patient care issues at the nurse-patient level. This has resulted in the successful implementation of many unit-based QA programs. However, the importance of having the units participate in a program evaluation process is not fully recognized. Unit-based program evaluations are valuable aids for QA managers' decision-making. We must ask ourselves

1. How do we create forums for all units to discuss their accomplishments, areas to improve, and plans for accomplishing necessary changes?
2. How do we identify the high-volume needs of our nursing units?
3. How do we provide a system of sharing successful problem-solving methods from unit to unit?

The answer is to make the program evaluation process an important program component.

The Richards Management Model has potential for unit-based application. A program evaluation workshop was given for all units at the author's institution. The medical-surgical division were grouped separately from the specialty divisions. This increased sharing and participation. It was amazing to hear and witness so many nursing managers and nurses from the units discussing their recognition of the need to involve all levels of staff in the unit's problem-solving process. They actually applied the program evaluation process to their units. This provided them with structure, focus, and confidence that they were moving in the right direction.

The combined results of using the program evaluation process for the unit-based program can have phenomenal results in terms of the overall program's effectiveness and attainment of program objectives. There is greater ownership and participation in unit-based QA programs. The nursing staff are highly motivated because they share their recommendations and are involved in the evaluation process. They implement various projects on their units to assist the program's effectiveness and efficiency. An example of such motivation is the nursing staff's development of a QA self-learning module to increase understanding of the QA process and establish peer review systems. Such involvement ensures that successful problem-solving methods will be developed and reflects ongoing program improvement. The nursing staff have a great deal of pride in their system and are very confident of its effectiveness.

CONCLUSION

To survive and prosper, hospitals must demonstrate their ability to improve and maintain quality of care. The program evaluation process must be viewed as a vital resource for all health care managers to use in decision making and in maintaining control of care via QA programs. QA is the essential factor in accreditation decisions, competition, and satisfied consumers—our self-insurance for survival.

REFERENCES

Clemenhagen, C., & Champagne, F. (1986). Quality assurance as part of program evaluation. *Quality Review Bulletin, 12*, 383.

Culp, B., Gormaere, N.D., & Miller, M.E. (1985). Risk management: An integral part of quality assurance. In C. Meisenheimer (Ed.), *Quality assurance, A complete guide to effective programs.* Gaithersburg, MD: Aspen Publishers.

Donabedian, A. (1980). *Explorations in quality assessment and monitoring: Vol. 1. The definition of quality and approaches to its assessment.* Ann Arbor, MI: Health Administration Press.

Loveridge, C.E. (1983). Quality assurance in nursing: The state of the art. In R.D. Luke, J.C. Krueger, & R.E. Modrow (Eds.), *Organization and change in health care quality assurance.* Gaithersburg, MD: Aspen Publishers.

Mehnert, T. (1985). The reassessment process: Key to a meaningful quality assurance program. *Quarterly Review Bulletin, 11*, 127–131.

Michnich, M.E., Shortell, S., & Richardson, W.C. (1981). Program evaluation: Resource for decision making. *Health Care Management Review, 6*, 25–35.

Schriven, M. (1967). The methodology of evaluation. In R. Tyler, R. Gagne, & M. Scriven (Eds.), *Perspectives on Curriculum Evaluation* (pp. 39–83). Chicago: Rand-McNally.

Scott, W.R. (1983). Managing professional work: Three models of control for health organization. In R.D. Luke, J.C. Krueger, & R.E. Modrow (Eds.), *Organization and change in health care quality assurance.* Gaithersburg, MD: Aspen Publishers.

Shanahan, M. (1983). The quality assurance standard of the JCAH: A rational approach to patient care evaluation. In R.D. Luke, J.C. Krueger, & R.E. Modrow (Eds.), *Organization and change in health care quality assurance.* Gaithersburg, MD: Aspen Publishers.

Sheldon, A., & Barrett, D. (1977). The Janus principle. *Health Care Management Review, 2*, 77–87.

Shortell, S.M., & Richardson, W.C. (1987). *Health Program Evaluation.* St. Louis: CV Mosby.

Smeltzer, C.H. (1985). Evaluating program effectiveness. In C.G. Meisenheimer (Ed.), *Quality assurance, a complete guide to effective programs.* Gaithersburg, MD: Aspen Publishers.

Wilson, C. (1984). Program evaluation: Theory, method and practice. In P. Schroeder & R. Maibusch (Eds.), *Nursing quality assurance, unit based approach.* Gaithersburg, MD: Aspen Publishers.

13

Toward a Quality Alliance with the Hospital Board

Madeline Musante Wake, PhD, RN, Assistant Professor and Director of Continuing Education and Outreach, Marquette University College of Nursing, Milwaukee, Wisconsin; Vice-Chairperson, Board of Directors, Trinity Memorial Hospital, Cudahy, Wisconsin

Nurse specialists in quality assurance (QA) are often asked to make verbal or written reports to the hospital board of directors. Such reporting may be seen as a mechanical activity, a challenge, or a confrontation. It is, in fact, an opportunity to participate in the strategic improvement of the organization. In order to participate fully, it is important to understand the role and functions of the board and the board's concern for quality.

ROLES AND FUNCTIONS OF THE HOSPITAL BOARD

The hospital board of directors "represents the corporate leadership and ownership. That is to say, the hospital board is ultimately responsible for the institution, the protection of its assets, and the quality of the services provided to its patients" (Umbdenstock, 1983, p. 11). Witt (1987) stated that hospital boards were previously called "boards of trustees," connoting stewardship, but are now commonly called "boards of directors," a term connoting a more active role equal to that of boards in business and industry.

Mott (1984) has detailed the four essential functional areas in hospital governance as community relations, strategic planning, financing, and QA. In its *Hospital Trustee Development Program* (1979), the American Hospital Association specified nine board functions. Three functions echoed by Mott were long-range planning, ensuring financial stability, and community relations. Additional functions were establishing board procedures, establishing goals and policies, and selecting and evaluating the chief executive officer. The three remaining functions could be included under the broad category of QA; they were to "monitor and evaluate plans and programs to ensure that they meet hospital goals and policies and the objectives of the long range plan," "approve selection of the medical staff and ensure that it is properly organized," and "provide a process for evaluation of

all phases of hospital performance, including the quality of its medical staff''
(pp. 6, 8). In order to better understand the board, it is useful to focus on its broad
functions.

Community Relations

Directors play a key role in interpreting their hospital to the community and
community needs to hospital administration. With increasing frequency, they are
assisted in this function by community advisory boards who concentrate on public
relations and fund raising. The board ensures that mechanisms are in place to
assess the health care needs of the community, alter programs in line with these
needs, and promulgate the contributions and positive impact of the hospital.

Strategic Planning

Through strategic planning, directors analyze the relationship between the
hospital and its external environment, including societal, economic, and regulatory factors. Based on their analysis and in concert with hospital administration
and clinical leadership, they plot a course for the hospital with an emphasis on its
mission, while balancing concerns for service and economic viability.

Financial Assurance

Directors ensure that there are effective systems in place for the revenue
generation, cash management, and resource utilization, which result in financial
soundness. They approve major expenditures as well as related loans. On a regular
basis, they compare actual revenue and expenditures with budgeted amounts and
ask for justifications of variance.

Quality Assurance

In an American Hospital Association board orientation booklet, Umbdenstock
(1983) has compared the hospital's QA program to quality control systems in
business and industry. He specified the five hospital QA areas as (1) medical staff
appointment, (2) facilities and equipment safety and utilization review,
(3) patient care evaluation, (4) risk management, and (5) continuing education.
    While hospital QA is a complex matter and involves all hospital employees and
members of the medical staff, the legal and ultimate responsibility for hospital

quality lies with the board of directors. This responsibility was illustrated in the landmark case of *Darling v. Charleston Community Memorial Hospital* (1965), in which the court ruled against the hospital and held it responsible for the quality of care provided by its medical staff. It is clear that directors have every reason to attend to quality issues.

The Joint Commission on Accreditation of Healthcare Organizations (Joint Commission) (1989) charges the board with the responsibility for maintaining quality patient care and requires board oversight of the QA program. As with its financial responsibility, the board does not manage the QA process. Rather, directors ensure that a system has been designed and implemented, that meaningful reports are generated, and that resulting information is used in decision making.

According to James Parsek, who is associate director of the department of standards of the Joint Commission,

> Explicit in the Joint Commission standards and required characteristics for the governing body is the requirement that the governing body assure that mechanisms are in place and used to assure that all persons who provide patient care in the hospital, whether subject to the medical staff credentialing and privileging or not, are competent to perform their duties. At the time of reappointment for persons subject to the medical staff credentialing and privileging mechanism and at the time of evaluation for all others, information from the quality assurance program is to be used in determining either reappointment or, in the case of persons who work under a job description, the ability to continue performing assigned duties. The governing body must be made aware of this information for each individual with clinical privileges and at least annually in a written summary report for all persons who work under a job description. Additionally the governing body is responsible for assuring that a planned, systematic and on-going program of quality assurance exists in the organization, that when problems or opportunities to improve are found effective actions are taken, and that improvements are sustained.
>
> The step beyond an effective quality assurance program is an emphasis on continued quality improvement. While quality assurance has tended to focus on making sure we do well what we do now, improvement focuses on the question: "Even though we're doing well now, how can we do better tomorrow?" The governing body, managerial, medical staff, nursing, and other clinical leaders must take a clear lead in focusing on quality improvement. (personal communication, November 7, 1989)

According to a 1989 survey conducted for the journal *Hospitals*, 51.3% of hospital chief executive officers want governing boards to be more active in ensuring quality of care (Koska, 1989). This need has been reflected in contingency data from the Joint Commission. Bohr and Taylor (1989) reported that in 1988, 23% of hospitals surveyed received contingencies (notification that accreditation was dependent upon correction) "for the board's failure to adequately evaluate QA information" (p. 15). Strategies to strengthen the board's efforts in QA are the formation of a standing board committee on quality or addition of a director as a member of the hospital QA committee.

As emphasis on cost containment and efficiency increases, directors are aware of and concerned about the quality consequences of cost reduction. Yet for many, the concern is vague and its analysis inscrutable. Board members are more aware of indicators of fiscal soundness than of appropriate indicators of patient health outcome following a brief hospitalization. When the board is informed of a decision to reduce staff in order to lower costly care hours per patient day, directors would also like to know the measures that indicate safety and nursing effectiveness and that a system exists to monitor them.

Changing Role of the Hospital Board

The role of the hospital board is undergoing substantive change (Griffith, 1988; Kovner, 1985; Shortell, 1989). As health care institutions adopt the corporate model, the board role is moving closer to that of governing boards in industry. In the past, trustees were chosen to represent community stakeholders. From being a position of honor and linkages, the director position is shifting to one of focused effort and expertise in providing strategic direction. With this shift, there is a sharper contrast between management and governance. The role of the board is governance, that is, setting strategic direction, ensuring compliance with mission and fiscal goals, and ratifying policy.

THE LEADERSHIP TRIAD FOR HOSPITALS

The leadership team in business and industry is comprised of owners and managers or governing boards and administration. One major difference between corporate and hospital organizations is the presence in the hospital of a large and powerful group who are predominantly not employees—the medical staff. Persons socialized into health care accept the structure of medical staff relations. Many directors have their roots in other than health care organizations and find the power of the medical staff perplexing, as may be shown by an analogy drawn from a non–health care situation. One can imagine the impact on the airline industry if the pilots were to be an independently organized group connected to one or more companies through bylaws rather than employment contracts. What would occur if the only way an individual could purchase an airplane ticket were through the pilot? What would happen if the pilot were to decide the class of service the passenger received, with no impact on the pilot's income? Owners and managers of the company would create new collaborative relationships or search for means to introduce incentives into the pilots' reward system.

The traditional leadership triad for hospitals has been administration, the governing board, and the medical staff. There has been tension and at times animosity among these three powers. However, in the current health care crisis, collaboration is essential. This mandate for collaboration extends to quality concerns. Shortell and LoGerfo (1981) found that overall medical staff participation in hospital decision making (as measured by membership of the chief of staff and other physicians on the hospital board) was the single most important variable associated with lower standardized mortality ratios from acute myocardial infarction.

When calling for more nurses to be included on hospital boards of directors, Smith (1986) stated that "nurses need direct access, indeed membership, on hospital boards to represent themselves in a publicly responsible manner and to see that nursing resources are committed within justly accountable bounds" (p. 48). She noted proposals for setting up self-governing nursing staffs that, like medical staffs, would report directly to the board.

Whether or not that ever occurs, the value of the nursing perspective in hospital leadership is becoming more accepted. Shortell (1985) has noted that a nurse as part of the top hospital management team can focus the organization on the priority of patient care. The leadership triad of the hospital may evolve to one of board, administration, and clinical leadership, the latter including medical and nursing staff.

QUALITY REPORTS TO THE BOARD

As the board receives regular financial reports, so it should regularly be informed of quality data. More and more boards have a committee to oversee the quality system. Operational monitoring is a hospital staff function, but oversight belongs to the board. In this regard, it is appropriate for the administrator to direct the QA coordinator to send copies to the board quality review committee of plans to monitor quality related to a new, changed, or problematic program or service.

When the QA coordinator presents to the board or board committee for the first time, it is useful to establish a climate for alliance by acknowledging the board's responsibility for quality care; by giving a brief overview of the coordinator role, the QA program, and planned reports; and by offering assistance. Such assistance may include provision of detailed information on a selected problem, suggestions of alternatives for meeting a new criterion, or offers to track the patient care impact of organizational changes.

Singleton and Nail (1986) offered suggestions to nurse executives for developing relationships with hospital boards of directors. Some of these suggestions may be valuable to the QA coordinator who gives reports to the full board or its committee. Singleton and Nail emphasized the mandate for confidentiality of board business, the need to refrain from disagreements with administration during meetings, and the value of brief summary reports with prepared detail available if requested.

For regular presentations to the board, the QA coordinator should submit a brief abstract of salient points (with detailed attachment if requested) to be sent out with the meeting agenda. Any verbal report should be brief and allow time for questions. The meeting of the board or board committee is not the time to work out problems with the chief executive officer or chief of the medical staff. Rather, such problems should be analyzed cooperatively beforehand and a data-based recommendation or a considered dilemma presented to the board.

In order to satisfy its accountability for oversight of QA, the board needs regular, substantive reports. Reports may be classified as program evaluation, ongoing quality indicators, and summary quality indicators. On an annual basis the total QA program should be evaluated and the evaluation summary, recommendations, and plans for improvement presented to the board.

Regular Quality Reports

Financial reports are submitted to the board monthly. The written reports include a comparison of budget with actual expenses and revenue and related statistics, such as average daily census and number of outpatient visits. During any regular meeting, directors may question significant budget-to-actual variances or ask the reason for an increase or decline in census. Such reports are essential for the board, to ensure financial soundness. Likewise, quality reports are essential.

Monthly quality reports to the board may be limited to a few significant elements presented in a format that facilitates comparison with past performance as well as with a standard or the institutional norm. Selected quantitative data such as nosocomial infection rate may be combined with qualitative data such as formal complaints. Each hospital board may individualize the monthly report to meet its needs for quality oversight. One list of quality elements that could be routinely presented to the board is displayed in Table 13-1.

Annual Quality Summary

In addition to monthly reports, the board should receive an annual compilation of quality data. Some elements for such a report were proposed by MacStravic

Table 13-1 Monthly Quality Report to Board

serious incidents, patient/visitor impact, corrective action
serious patient, physician, and employee complaints, investigation, follow-up
number of transfers to other hospitals initiated for other than unavailable service
number of delinquent records, actions taken
unscheduled returns to surgery
readmission before 7 and 30 days postdischarge
nosocomial infection rate

(1989) in his value-based performance report, the Values Accounting and Reporting System. He noted the importance of soft data, such as public reputation and patient satisfaction, to complement quantitative data. An annual quality report may include data on patient satisfaction, community impact, medical staff, employees, and care outcomes. Goran, Roberts, and Rodak (1976) have written that "the hospital represents a relatively closed system in which the professional staff is organized, continuing education is an ongoing process, patient health problems are relatively circumscribed, and data on the care provided are readily retrievable" (p. 62). The QA coordinator or a member of the top administrative team can take advantage of existing data to develop a meaningful and comprehensive annual summary report for the board. Data elements for such a report are displayed in Table 13-2.

These data may be drawn from many sources. For example, patient satisfaction and community impact data may be collected by the marketing or public relations department. The medical executive committee, medical staff office, and medical records department can provide data on medical staff. Employee data can be collected by the personnel department. Indicators with both cost and quality components, such as payments denied or transfers to other facilities, can be provided by the finance department.

In addition to compilations of existing data, concern for more comprehensive measures of quality and appropriateness may necessitate the collection of new data. Donabedian (1987) discussed studies of entire episodes of care and studies of the effects of prospective payment on quality. He emphasized that confining quality assessment to the period of hospitalization is too limiting. With the emphasis upon shortened length of stay, the true outcomes of care are not obvious until after the patient has been discharged. On a selective basis, patients from one of the leading diagnosis-related groups (DRGs) for a hospital could be studied postdischarge. Such episode-of-illness studies would yield data on health status outcomes and cost shifting, which could be used to improve inpatient care.

Table 13-2 Annual Hospital Quality Summary

- Patient satisfaction
  1. satisfaction questionnaires: percent of total patients represented and results and follow-up
  2. transfers into and out of hospital
  3. review of serious patient complaints
  4. improvement strategies
- Quality and appropriateness of care
  1. nosocomial infection rate
  2. unscheduled returns to surgery
  3. readmissions before 7, 15, and 30 days after discharge
  4. mortality
  5. percent of deaths presented for mortality review
  6. severity-adjusted mortality
  7. payment denials and changes
  8. episode of illness study
- Medical staff
  1. total number per staff category
  2. percent board certified
  3. number of physicians reviewed for privileges: appointment, promotion, reappointment; number accepted/number denied
  4. number of new claims against physicians
  5. average time for completion of delinquent records
  6. physician complaints and resignations
  7. improvement strategies
- Employees
  1. total number and numbers by categories
  2. percent of new employees having orientation program
  3. turnover rates of selected groups
  4. performance appraisal system and summary of ratings
  5. mandatory inservice education programs (percent attendance)
  6. grievances and employee welfare problems
  7. improvement strategies
- Community
  1. number of community education programs
  2. outreach to schools, industries
  3. number of individuals reached
  4. contribution to indigent care

REPRESENTING NURSING TO THE BOARD

Nurse executives and nurse QA coordinators who attend meetings of the board or board committees represent nursing in actions and reports. This representation is not of the nursing department alone, but of the entire discipline. Often nurses perceive that the board is disinterested in nursing and that directors focus quality concerns on medicine. Interest in nursing may be enhanced by demonstrating the relationship between the community image of hospital quality and patient satisfaction with nursing care. Medical credentialing has been and is now a major board responsibility. However, recent Joint Commission standards make it clear that the board must also ensure the quality of nurses employed. This new emphasis requires education of the board about nursing.

Directors are aware of the fact that nurses comprise a large segment of hospital employees, but often they know little about the nursing profession. In the second volume of its *Hospital Trustee Development Program*, the American Hospital Association (1981) addressed the role of the governing board in issues concerning nursing. Boards were advised to (1) examine joint physician-nurse practice models, (2) encourage physician understanding of nursing issues, and (3) support initiatives to improve the professional satisfaction of hospital nurses.

Information on the nature and value of nursing can be included in reports or support for projected changes. Directors would benefit from reading the research support for the statement by the National Commission on Nursing Implementation Project (1988) that a "fuller and more appropriate use of nurses in providing health services would allow containment of health care costs without sacrificing quality" (p. 8).

For example, Brooten and associates (1988) designed a model for nurse specialist home care of patients following early discharge. The model incorporated tracking of quality of care through patient outcome and cost data. When the model was tested with very low birth weight infants (Brooten et al., 1986), the early discharge group was discharged an average of 11 days earlier, with a mean savings of $18,560 per case and without significant differences in patient outcomes when compared to the control group.

Research findings also address the importance of nurse-physician relationships. Knaus, Draper, Wagner, and Zimmerman (1986) compared the predicted and actual death rates in 5030 patients cared for in intensive care units of 13 tertiary care hospitals. They found significant differences in actual to predicted death ratios related to the interaction and communication between physicians and nurses. This study provides support for the worth of joint practice committees and collaborative models for intensive care unit direction.

Many directors are concerned about the nursing shortage. Prescott (1989) reframed the problem as a shortage of professional nursing practice. She contended that the hospital organization constrains and blocks the professional practice capabilities of nurses. She stated, "Given the need for a more cost-effective delivery system in the hospital, the continued existence of a system that underuses the knowledge, skill, and experience of the nation's largest health manpower source is counterproductive" (p. 441). Her work could be used to lend support to plans for changes in nurse utilization.

Indicators of Nursing Quality

The selection of indicators of nursing quality communicates much about the nature of nursing. Loveridge (1983) contended, "It will never be possible to develop valid measurements of quality if the elements of nursing practice are not properly conceptualized and made more explicit" (p. 259).

Measurement of the outcomes of nursing care is difficult due to the complexity and holistic nature of nursing practice, as well as the fact that many health outcomes are the result of collaborative efforts of patients, physicians, nurses, and often other health professionals. However, a system designed to ensure quality cannot be limited to structure and process standards. Outcome standards and measures are essential. Brett (1989) listed categories of measurable outcomes, including patient satisfaction, knowledge, compliance and perceptions; functional, clinical, or psychoemotional health status; and discharge readiness of the patient. While the system of measuring nursing outcomes is imperfect at present, there is a need to select nursing outcome indicators for monitoring and reporting to the board.

Seeking a way to establish the cost-effectiveness of quality nursing care, Barrett (1988) developed and tested a mechanism for using raw data from the HEW— Medicus Nursing Process Methodology to compute quality scores for DRGs. Linked to a DRG instead of a nursing unit, such quality scores could be used to evaluate the relationship of quality nursing care and length of hospital stay. In one hospital, professional nursing case management has been applied to maintain quality while converting DRG money losers to revenue sources (Ethridge & Lamb, 1989).

There is a need for improvement in individual nurse accountability for given outcomes. Medicine can tie individual physician accountability to such indicators as infection or complication rate, return to surgery, and readmission within 30 days. However, most current nursing systems do not capture individual nurse accountability for self-care knowledge upon discharge, or the presence of postoperative respiratory complications. In the nursing minimum data set (NMDS), Werley (1987) suggested the individual nurse provider be identified as one of the several standard data elements to be captured by information systems. In piloting the NMDS, that element was the least used. However, H.H. Werley (personal communication, September 15, 1989) stated that the element would be retained and that she expected it to be used in the future.

Other Nursing Concerns of the Board

In addition to the nursing shortage, physician-nurse relationships, and other topics already addressed, there are other nursing issues that concern directors. For one, directors are concerned with the quality as well as the cost consequences of heavy use of supplemental staff. Another area of concern is granting of special staff privileges to nurses. For this role, it is unclear if an advanced degree or credential, such as specialty certification, should be required.

CONCLUSION

As health care leaves a decade of preoccupation with cost containment and enters a decade of seeing cost-effective quality as a differential advantage in marketing an institution (Nelson & Goldstein, 1989), if not a mandate for survival, those invested in the future of a hospital must join forces. The QA coordinator can consciously promote an alliance of the board, administration, and clinical leadership focused on the shared mission of an institutionally defined commitment to quality patient care.

REFERENCES

American Hospital Association. (1979). *Hospital trustee development program* (Vol. 1). Chicago: Author.

American Hospital Association. (1981). *Hospital trustee development program* (Vol. 2). Chicago: Author.

Barrett, E.A. (1988). Measuring quality of nursing care for DRGs using the HEW-Medicus nursing process methodology. In O.L. Strickland & C.F. Waltz (Eds.), *Measurement of nursing outcomes: Vol. 2. Measuring nursing performance* (pp. 154–177). New York: Springer.

Bohr, D., & Taylor, D. (1989). QA orientation and reporting: Problem areas for boards. *Trustee, 42*(9), 15, 27.

Brett, J.L. (1989). Outcome indicators of quality care. In B. Henry, C. Arndt, M. DiVencenti, & A. Marriner-Tomey (Eds.), *Dimensions of nursing administration* (pp. 353–369). St. Louis: Blackwell.

Brooten, D., Brown, L.P., Munro, B.H., York, R., Cohen, S.M., Roncoli, M., & Hollingsworth, A. (1988). Early discharge and specialist transitional care. *Image, 20*, 64–68.

Brooten, D., Kumar, S., Brown, L., Butts, P., Finkler, S., Bakewell-Sachs, S., Gibbons, A., & Delivoria-Papadopoulos, M. (1986). A randomized clinical trial of early hospital discharge and home followup of very low birthweight infants. *New England Journal of Medicine, 315*, 934–939.

Darling v. Charleston Community Memorial Hospital, 33 Ill.2d 326, 211 N.E.2d 253 (1965).

Donabedian, A. (1987). Commentary on some studies of the quality of care. *Health Care Financing Review, 8* (Annual suppl.), 75–85.

Ethridge, P., & Lamb, G.S. (1989). Professional nursing case management improves quality, access, and costs. *Nursing Management, 20*(3), 30–35.

Goran, M.J., Roberts, J.S., & Rodak, J. (1976). Regulating the quality of hospital care—an analysis of the issues pertinent to national health insurance. In R.H. Egdahl & P.M. Gertman (Eds.), *Quality assurance in health care* (p. 62). Gaithersburg, MD: Aspen Publishers, Inc.

Griffith, J.R. (1988). Voluntary hospitals: Are trustees the solution? *Hospital & Health Services Administration, 33*, 295–310.

Joint Commission on Accreditation of Healthcare Organizations. (1989). *Accreditation manual for hospitals*. Chicago: Author.

Knaus, W.A., Draper, E.A., Wagner, D.P., & Zimmerman, J.E. (1986). An evaluation of outcome from intensive care in major medical centers. *Annals of Internal Medicine, 104*, 410–418.

Koska, M.T. (1989). CEO—board relationships: An update. *Hospitals, 63*(7), 38–42.

Kovner, A.R. (1985). Improving the effectiveness of hospital governing boards. *Frontiers of Health Services Management, 2*, 4–33.

Loveridge, C.E. (1983). Quality assurance in nursing: The state of the art. In R.D. Luke, J.C. Krueger, & R.E. Modrow (Eds.), *Organization and change in health care quality assurance* (pp. 253–261). Gaithersburg, MD: Aspen Publishers.

MacStravic, R.S. (1989). Tracking hospital performance. *Trustee, 42*(6), 15, 27.

Mott, B.J.F. (1984). *Trusteeship and the future of community hospitals*. Chicago: American Hospital Publishing.

National Commission on Nursing Implementation Project. (1988). *The nation's nurses: A credible profession doing an incredible job*. Milwaukee, WI: Author.

Nelson, C.W., & Goldstein, A.S. (1989). Health care quality: The new marketing challenge. *Health Care Management Review, 14*, 87–95.

Prescott, P.A. (1989). Shortage of professional nursing practice: A reframing of the shortage problem. *Heart & Lung, 18*, 436–443.

Shortell, S.M. (1985). High-performing health care organizations: Guidelines for the pursuit of excellence. *Hospital & Health Services Administration, 30*(4), 7–35.

Shortell, S.M. (1989). New directions in hospital governance. *Hospital & Health Services Administration, 34*(1), 7–23.

Shortell, S.M., & LoGerfo, J.P. (1981). Hospital medical staff organization and quality of care: Results for myocardial infarction and appendectomy. *Medical Care, 19*, 1041–1055.

Singleton, E.K., & Nail, F.C. (1986). Developing relationships with the board of directors. *Journal of Nursing Administration, 16*(1), 37–42.

Smith, E.D. (1986). Nurse trustee: Getting power over policy. *Nursing Management, 17*(7), 48, 50.

Umbdenstock, R.J. (1983). *So You're on the Hospital Board*. Chicago: American Hospital Publishing.

Werley, H.H. (1987). Nursing diagnosis and the nursing minimum data set. In A.M. McLane (Ed.), *Classification of nursing diagnoses: Proceedings of the seventh conference* (pp. 21–36). St. Louis: CV Mosby.

Witt, J.A. (1987). *Building a better hospital board*. Ann Arbor, MI: Health Administration Press.

14

Evolving Approaches to Quality Improvement

Patricia Schroeder, MSN, RN, Nursing Quality Consultant, Quality Care
Concepts, Inc., Thiensville, Wisconsin

Traditional quality assurance (QA) programs have earned the reputation of being negatively oriented, tedious in their process, and focused predominantly on documentation. At best they have made little impact on clinical practice. At worst they have divested practitioners of any curiosity about clinical improvement through quality programs and have wasted untold dollars in precious health care resources that could have been better spent. Many health care organizations, however, have begun to take a new look at QA programs. America's increasing quality orientation, along with the need to improve processes in light of fiscal constraints and changing expectations of external reviewing/accrediting agencies, has shifted attention from QA to quality improvement (QI) philosophies.

QA, as a label, suggested more than it ever really achieved. It suggested that assessment and measurement of quality were not the end of the process. One needed to take actions to ensure a given level of care. Given the complexity of health care organizations, human systems, and their interactions, however, this assurance was really never a guarantee. The process stopped too often with identification of the negative or, at best, achievement of the mediocre. Dennis O'Leary, president of the Joint Commission on Accreditation of Healthcare Organizations (Joint Commission), states, "In retrospect, the word 'assurance' was an unfortunate semantic selection. Quality, of course, could never be assured. Rather, it could at best only be improved" (O'Leary, 1990, p. 2).

Patterson (1990) describes the evolution in thought that affected quality programs espoused by the Joint Commission. She states that health care has gone from quality audit, to quality assessment, to quality assurance, to quality improvement. Each step built on the philosophy and experience of the past. Quality improvement will be increasingly emphasized by the Joint Commission in their standards for health care organizations (O'Leary, 1990).

Many initials are used today to describe various quality programs: QA, quality assurance; QI, quality improvement; CQI, continuous quality improvement; TQI, total quality improvement; TQM, total quality management; TQS, total quality systems; and more. Whereas it is likely that when originally coined, these phrases differentiated specific ideologies, today, right or wrong, they are often used interchangeably.

QI philosophies are based on several consistent premises. There must be a clarification of and vigilant attention to the true mission of the organization. Those carrying out the work of the organization must be empowered to measure and improve the process and product of their work. There must be an unleashing of creativity and flexibility to better meet the needs of internal and external customers. Internal customers are those coworkers within the organization who are dependent on aspects of your work to successfully complete their own. External customers are those outside of the organization to whom your product or service is delivered or from whom some payment is received.

The term "quality improvement" suggests that quality can always be made better. Rather than working to achieve an arbitrary, specific level of performance reflecting an established norm, one should compare oneself to oneself over time, with the goal being continuous improvement.

The role of leadership is vital in organizations implementing a QI approach. Leaders must set the tone for the organization's commitment to quality and its mission. They must be visible proponents of the quality message—must support, nurture, demand, and reward quality. Whereas traditional QA programs received little attention from hospital leaders, success in QI programs can only be achieved through focus on and attention from those in leadership roles. Peters and Austin (1985) summarize this point by stating, "Any device to maintain quality can be of value. But all devices are valuable if managers—at all levels—are living the quality message, paying attention to quality, spending time on it as evidenced by their calendars. And if managers, at all levels, understand that no matter where the technology leads, quality comes from people (starting in the mail room) who care and are committed" (p. 115).

Innovation is also considered an essential ingredient in QI programs. Evolving science and technology were historically responsible for innovations in health care. Traditional practices and processes have been considered almost sacred. Today's view of innovation is based on small starts and autonomous or decentralized approaches (Peters, 1987, p. 53). Innovations must stem from those carrying out the work of the organization, rather than solely from research and development departments. Everyone is encouraged to play a role in innovating improvements, with emphasis placed on better meeting the needs of internal or external customers, creating a better product or more efficient process, and increasing productivity and cost-effectiveness.

While many have contributed to the evolution of philosophies and approaches to QI, three names consistently appear in the literature. Deming, Juran, and Crosby have been touted as the best-known names in the quality business, "the real leaders—the big three who have achieved guru status" (Oberle, 1990, p. 47).

W. Edwards Deming, an engineer and statistician, has been credited for his role in bringing the quality message to Japan to aid in post-World War II reconstruction. Through his efforts, the Japanese worked to create an industrial foundation as well as a society focused attentively on quality and QI (Walton, 1986). He is also considered the parent of statistical quality control, most specifically self-inspection by workers on the line (Peters & Austin, 1985, p. 118). Deming established 14 points for QI, which have evolved from his international work. These are described in his seminal work *Out of the Crisis* (Deming, 1986). The points have been applied in a variety of industries, to a lesser extent in service industries such as health care. Given that the service sector now employs 75% of American workers, these applications are critical to many both within and outside of health care (Peters, 1987, p. 7). Gillem (1988) applies these 14 points to hospitals, based on the work being carried out by Hospital Corporation of America (HCA). Kosta (1990) further describes the use of Deming's principles at one HCA hospital, Parkview Episcopal Medical Center.

Joseph M. Juran was also involved in early work in Japan's industrial rebuilding. He emphasized the importance of incorporating managers into the pursuit of quality. He is also credited with the concept of attending to the needs of internal customers as well as to those of external customers. Juran has created a structured approach to what he labels the "quality trilogy"—quality planning, quality control, and QI (Juran, 1988).

Philip B. Crosby gained prominence following the publication of his book *Quality Is Free* in 1979. Crosby provides a less technically oriented approach to QI, addressing attitudes and behaviors among people. His 14-step approach to QI has also precipitated many positive results in organizations around the world.

Oberle (1990) states that rather than working to identify distinctions between ideologies, it is most beneficial to seek their commonalities to guide implementation in an organization. All emphasize the importance of attention to quality by organizational leaders, empowerment of workers, measurement of quality parameters, and the need for continuous improvement. He suggests specific techniques of one or the other might be adopted based on what best meets the needs of and fits with the organization.

Holpp (1989) states that irrespective of the ideology, QI is neither easy nor guaranteed with a quick fix. QI approaches, while sounding logical, worthwhile, and achievable, are only successful with intensive efforts. Total redesign of the workplace and planned shifting of organizational culture are massive undertakings that require commitment, resources, and time to achieve.

Hoernschmeyer (1989) inter-relates quality improvement philosophies and approaches as he describes the four cornerstones of excellence for organizations today. He states that excellence requires (1) a quality context and culture that shapes and guides the work of the organization; (2) the empowerment of people with information, resources, and support; (3) intense and continuous communication about planned directions, problems, and outcomes; and (4) continuous identification and destruction of barriers to people's performance. These essential components create a solid foundation for quality within an organization. They also speak to an approach to quality very different from that with which we have become familiar in health care.

The humanization of the quality initiative has been a most welcome benefit in the shift from QA to QI. Rather than looking to identify problems and convey blame, we seek opportunities to improve. Rather than blindly holding to the rules, we seek to innovate. Rather than working to keep people in line, we look for ways to generate energy and excitement. The QI agenda is one that encourages people to find better ways to carry out their roles. For nurses, who have long proclaimed their commitment to patients, the implementation of QI methods is proving to be a valuable opportunity. It is taking the knowledge that nurses have about patient needs and perceptions and beginning to incorporate it into organizational change. QI holds the potential of improving patient care in a way that QA never did. By learning from the 40 years of experience of others using QI ideas and techniques, we can greatly assist in the generation of commitment to quality in this complex arena called health care.

REFERENCES

Crosby, P. (1979). *Quality is free*. New York, McGraw-Hill.

Deming, W.E. (1986). *Out of the crisis*. Cambridge, MA: MIT Center for Advanced Engineering Study.

Gillem, T.R. (1988). Deming's 14 points and hospital quality: Responding to the consumer's demand for the best value health care. *Journal of Nursing Quality Assurance, 2*, 70–78.

Hoernschmeyer, D. (1989). The four cornerstones of excellence. *Quality Progress, 22*, 37–40.

Holpp, L. (1989). 10 reasons why total quality is less than total. *Training, 26*, 93–103.

Juran, J.M. (1988). *Juran on planning for quality*. New York: Free Press.

Kosta, M.T. (1990). Adapting Deming's quality improvement ideas: A case study. *Hospitals, 64*, 58–62, 64.

Oberle, J. (1990). Quality gurus: The men and their message. *Training, 27*, 47–52.

O'Leary, D. (1990). President's column—CQI-A step beyond QA. *Joint Commission Perspectives, 10*, 2–3.

Patterson, C.H. (1990). Quality assurance, control and monitoring: The future role of information technology from the Joint Commission's perspective. *Computers in Nursing, 8*, 105–110.

Peters, T., & Austin, N. (1985). *A passion for excellence: The leadership difference*. New York: Warner Books.

Peters, T. (1987). *Thriving on chaos: Handbook for a management revolution*. New York: Harper & Row.

Walton, M. (1986). *The Deming management method*. New York: Dodd, Mead, & Co.

Index

215